THE GOOD NEWS ABOUT ASTHMA

DID YOU KNOW:

- Even the most severe asthma attack is rarely fatal.
- Most asthma patients can lead normal, active lives.
- Asthma is not caused by stress, although stress may be a contributory factor.
- Exercise can actually *improve* your condition.
- It is possible to fend off an attack before it occurs.
- Modern scientists believe asthma has a genetic cause and are working to unravel the genetic code.

These encouraging facts and much more are explored in this invaluable sourcebook that will show you how to recover your physical and emotional well-being and find the treatment that's best for you.

WHAT YOU CAN DO ABOUT ASTHMA

THE DELL MEDICAL LIBRARY

LEARNING TO LIVE WITH CHRONIC FATIGUE SYNDROME
LEARNING TO LIVE WITH CHRONIC IBS
RELIEF FROM CARPAL TUNNEL SYNDROME AND OTHER
REPETITIVE MOTION DISORDERS
RELIEF FROM CHRONIC ARTHRITIS PAIN
RELIEF FROM CHRONIC BACKACHE
RELIEF FROM CHRONIC HEADACHE
RELIEF FROM CHRONIC TMJ PAIN
WHAT WOMEN CAN DO ABOUT CHRONIC ENDOMETRIOSIS
WHAT WOMEN SHOULD KNOW ABOUT CHRONIC
INFECTIONS AND SEXUALLY TRANSMITTED DISEASES
WHAT WOMEN SHOULD KNOW ABOUT MENOPAUSE
WHAT YOU CAN DO ABOUT INFERTILITY
WHAT YOU CAN DO ABOUT DIABETES
WHAT YOU CAN DO ABOUT ASTHMA
WHAT YOU CAN DO ABOUT EPILEPSY

THE DELL MEDICAL LIBRARY

What You Can Do About
ASTHMA

Nathaniel Altman

*Foreword by David A. Mrazek, M.D.,
M.R.C. Psych.*

A LYNN SONBERG BOOK

Published by
Dell Publishing
a division of
Bantam Doubleday Dell Publishing Group, Inc.
1540 Broadway
New York, New York 10036

Medical research about asthma is ongoing and subject to interpretation. Although every effort has been made to include the most up-to-date and accurate information in this book, there can be no guarantee that what we know about these subjects today won't change with time. Readers should bear in mind that this book is not for the purpose of self-diagnosis or self-treatment, and they should consult appropriate medical professionals regarding all problems related to their health.

ISBN: 0-440-20641-3

Published by arrangement with Lynn Sonberg Book Services, 166 East 56 Street, New York, N.Y. 10022

Printed in the United States of America

Published simultaneously in Canada

October 1991

10 9 8 7 6 5 4 3

OPM

CONTENTS

ACKNOWLEDGMENTS

I would like to thank the following people who helped me in the successful completion of this book: Gary Alexander of the National Jewish Center for Immunology and Respiratory Medicine in Denver, for his generous assistance in obtaining important medical information and interviews with members of the staff. Special thanks go to David Mrazek, M.D., Bobby Sherman, Mike LaMothe, Dee Dee Valez, Jerry Gillette, Henry Milgram, M.D., Lana Selzer, and Malcolm Hill, Ph.D., at National Jewish for their valuable information and expertise.

I would also like to thank Thomas F. Plaut, M.D., for permission to use several of the drawings from his book *Children with Asthma,* and to the *British Medical Journal* for the use of drawings from the book *ABC of Asthma* (2nd ed.).

Finally, I want to express my deep gratitude to Sandra Chevalier for her encouragement and advice; to Sophie Aissen for providing a young person's perspective on asthma; and to Alexander Oland for his valuable suggestions, insights, and critique of the manuscript.

FOREWORD

While being director of pediatric psychiatry at the National Jewish Center for Immunology and Respiratory Medicine for more than a decade, I have had the opportunity to meet thousands of asthmatic children and come to know some of them very well indeed. I have also sat with their parents and have come to appreciate how difficult coping with severe asthma can be for the whole family. My clinical work at National Jewish has often involved helping these children to take a fresh look at their illness and to make a new and determined start toward a life that can be just as full as that of any child without asthma.

What You Can Do About Asthma presents practical information that is important for asthmatics and parents of asthmatics to learn about this illness. It is presented in a readable format and focuses on a wide range of medical and psychological considerations that are relevant for the management of the disease. It is timely in its medical presentation and comprehensive in its scope.

As one digests this volume, a recurrent theme is the importance of dismissing the "helplessness" myth that can affect so many asthmatics with this chronic illness. It is critical for adults, and especially children, to deal energetically with their symptoms rather than choosing to limit their activity. In fact, the overall quality of life that they eventually achieve is greatly dependent on the effectiveness of this effort.

Living with asthma involves understanding just what kind of triggers will aggravate the disease and working out strategies for dealing with them. The severity of asthma varies dramatically among individuals. More fortunate asthmatics have a mild, circumscribed form of the illness. They can hope to achieve a symptom-free status with relatively limited personal effort. However, some asthmatics have a severe form of the illness that is resistant to medication and is associated with severe respiratory attacks. This form of asthma requires the development of a partnership with a competent physician to monitor the pattern of attack carefully and to work out effective means of controlling these symptoms. It also requires sensitive psychological support and guidance in coping with the frightening and aggravating aspects of the asthma attacks. It is these difficult cases with which we have become most familiar at the National Jewish Center for Immunology and Respiratory Medicine.

The role played by emotions and psychological stress among asthma patients has always caused a great deal of confusion. Although emotions can be important factors in the disease, it does not follow that asthma is a strictly psychological illness. Clearly, asthma has genetic roots, and physical changes in the bronchial airways can be identified. However, it is also unquestionably true that intense emotional crises or chronic familial stressors can exacerbate the frequency and severity of asthmatic attacks. Coming to grips with the psychological aspects of the illness is particularly important, as it provides an opportunity to help families cope and thereby to reduce the severity of respiratory symptoms and emotional disability.

In summary, understanding one's illness is the first and most important step in learning how to manage it. The facts necessary to begin this process are contained within this volume. More importantly, abundant references and information are provided that will be useful to those asthmatics and their families who are motivated to find a way to live effectively with asthma.

DAVID A. MRAZEK, M.D., M.R.C. PSYCH.
Director, Pediatric Psychiatry
National Jewish Center for Immunology
and Respiratory Medicine

INTRODUCTION

Of all the chronic diseases of this century, asthma is one of the least understood. Although it affects approximately one person in twenty-five (and one child in ten!), often those of us who suffer from asthma feel alone and isolated. Asthma usually appears for the first time in children between two and five years of age, and it often disappears during the teenage years. Symptoms may then reappear during the adult years. Despite the medical advances in asthma diagnosis and treatment over the past few decades, asthma is on the increase. In large part this is because it is often incorrectly diagnosed and poorly managed. Visits to the hospital emergency room are up, and more people are dying from the disease every year. A growing percentage of these mortalities are children or young adults.

While physicians and medical researchers know what can trigger an asthma flare, they are not certain what actually causes people to be susceptible to the disease in the first place. Some people may experience only one or two asthma attacks throughout their lives, while others can suffer several during a twenty-four-hour period. An asthma flare can come on gradually or suddenly, it can take place while awake or asleep (in fact, about 30 percent of asthma attacks occur between three and six in the morning), and it can be triggered by such varied allergic factors as pollen, dust mites, or certain foods, or by nonallergenic factors such as cigarette smoke and other types of air pollution, cold air, laughter, exercise, or emotional stress. A mild asthma flare can last several minutes, while a more severe episode can last half a day or more.

In years past, most asthma therapies concentrated solely on the symptoms of the disease. In addition to being told to limit their physical activity, patients were routinely given powerful drugs such as epinephrine, which often produced severe, unpleasant side effects. They were taught that the best way to manage asthma was to slow down, keep quiet, try to cope as best they could, and consult the physician when symptoms got bad.

There are still no known cures for asthma. But there have been tremendous strides in asthma management during the past twenty years. Better diagnostic methods have been developed; the immune system reaction that triggers an attack has been identified; and safer, more effective medications have become available. Doctors are also more concerned with the *whole patient* rather than with symptoms alone. In addition to a careful physical evaluation, physicians take mental and emotional factors into account and how they can affect the patient's overall health. Family situation, diet, and exposure to trigger factors of asthma in the environment are also considered. Asthma sufferers are also being taught that the two keys to successful asthma management are *education* and *taking responsibility for one's health.* By learning about the dynamics of asthma and how it affects them personally, asthma sufferers learn how to control asthma flares and to prevent them from taking place as much as possible. They are encouraged to work with their physician as a team in learning how to monitor breathing, reduce exposure to trigger factors, and know when a doctor's care is needed. Despite myths that depict people with asthma as being condemned to a life of anxious suffering, physical limitation, and feelings of inferiority, most patients can learn to lead normal, active lives.

This book has been written expressly to provide the basic, most essential information about asthma to you as an asthma patient, your friends, and your family. My goal is not only to help you cope with asthma but also to help you thrive *in spite of it*. Using the latest medical knowledge from both the United States and Europe, this book is designed to offer you clear and accurate information about the nature of the disease, how it is diagnosed, and how it can be managed. Asthma is a complex and challenging disease, and to manage it properly requires a lifetime of study and understanding. This book is intended to be an important first step in this process. In the final analysis, knowledge and effective management skills will empower you, the asthma patient, to take charge of the disease, rather than having asthma control every aspect of your life.

The first part of this book provides a basic understanding of the disease, what triggers asthma attacks, and how asthma affects both children and adults. Part II notes what you should look for in a medical diagnosis, and explores the various ways that you can prevent and treat asthma with the help of both traditional medicine and complementary therapies. This doesn't mean that we are endorsing unorthodox treatments; rather, we are providing an overview for your information as a patient and health care consumer. We will also examine the ways in which we can effectively prevent and manage asthma attacks through environmental control, diet, and exercise.

Through a clear understanding about asthma, its triggers,

and its dynamics, you can work as a partner with your health care provider to develop strategies for effective and successful self-care. This will not only make your life easier and more fulfilling, it will also enable you to reach your highest health potential.

NATHANIEL ALTMAN
Brooklyn, New York
September 1990

PART I
UNDERSTANDING ASTHMA

WHAT IS ASTHMA?

Asthma is one of our most common chronic diseases, yet many people are not sure what it really is. Asthma is a disease that obstructs the airways and includes breathing difficulties, tightness in the chest, wheezing, and coughing. An important feature of asthma is that these symptoms can be reversed. During an asthma flare the muscles of the airways that connect your mouth and throat to the lungs tighten up. As the airways narrow, the flow of air both into and out of your lungs becomes obstructed.

Asthma affects over 11.2 million people in the United States alone, including 5 to 10 percent of all children, many of whom outgrow the disease by their midteens. Asthma patients spend over one billion dollars a year on medical treatment. This includes over twenty-seven million visits to the doctor's office, along with over four hundred thousand hospital admissions. Asthma patients also take a wide variety of asthma medications. Asthma is one of the major reasons for lost days and poor productivity at work and is the leading cause of absenteeism among children in primary and secondary school.

Asthma affects people of all ages, races, and cultural backgrounds. Medical science has not yet identified any specific "at risk" groups. However, a genetic factor may be involved: According to the British Medical Association, if you have at least one asthmatic parent, you are more likely to develop asthma than someone without asthmatic parents. This translates into a 25 percent chance of developing the disease if one of your parents suffered from asthma, and a 40 percent chance if both of your parents have had the disease. However, the risk depends in part on how severe your parent's asthma was. Some studies have shown that if you were breast-fed from birth, your chances of developing asthma may be reduced.

A curious side note: Asthma appears to be twice as likely to occur among boys under ten years of age as among girls.

IS ASTHMA PSYCHOSOMATIC?

Many asthma patients suffer from the widespread myth that asthma is psychosomatic in origin. Asthma is a genetic disease that always begins with the airway receptors and does not have its origin in the mind.

However, your emotions can play an important role in triggering an asthma attack. If you become angry or upset, you may *hyperventilate*—that is, you breathe both deeper and faster. If you are asthma-prone, this can, in turn, trigger an attack. Conscious relaxation and guided imagery can help you prevent and manage asthma symptoms.

Many asthma patients suffer from emotional problems brought about by having this chronic disease. In the first place, some suffer from the perception that they are somehow to blame for being sick, and they feel guilty for the inconvenience or expense their illness may cause. Secondly, they may be frustrated over the physical limitations that a disease such as asthma can place on their lives. Finally, some of the medications used to manage asthma have side effects that can lead to anxiety and depression. We'll discuss these medical and psychological factors in detail later on. Meanwhile, keep in mind that coping with any chronic illness can take an immense psychological toll. But people with asthma should rest assured that in psychological terms they are basically no different from anyone else.

THE MEDICAL EXPLANATION

When you experience an asthma attack, the airways of the lungs become narrower. At the same time, secretions of mucus may increase, the muscles in the walls of the airways can go into spasm, and the walls of the airways may swell up. Very often, all three of these problems occur during an attack.

A "trigger factor" is always involved when an asthma flare takes place. This can consist of an allergic response to ragweed, dust, or food coloring. It can also involve a reaction to cold, exercise, or stress. Sometimes there may be only one trigger factor present, although most patients respond to several. Trigger factors vary from person to person. They may also affect the same person at different times of the year.

Asthma symptoms vary dramatically. They can range from a slight tightening of the chest or occasional cough to intense feelings of breathlessness, coughing, and wheezing that can send you to the hospital emergency room. Severe asthma symptoms can be very frightening. During a moderate to severe attack, people with asthma often feel that they are fighting for every breath of air they take. As a result, they can experience extreme fear and panic to the point that they imagine they are going to suffocate to death. Although only 3 percent of individuals suffer from what doctors call "very severe" asthma (and the mortality rate from severe asthma is quite low compared to deaths from diabetes, heart disease, or cancer), such an attack can produce tremendous anxiety for both the sufferer and the family. A minor asthma flare can last for a few moments and suddenly disappear. Moderate to severe attacks can persist for several hours to a day or more.

If you suffer from asthma—or know someone who does— it's important to understand exactly what actually happens when an asthma flare takes place. Let's compare how the respiratory system functions in normal individuals and in those suffering from asthma symptoms.

THE NORMAL BREATH

Most of the time you take breathing completely for granted. However, when you run to catch a bus or feel that you're suffocating in a roomful of cigarette smoke, you become more aware of the breathing process. On rare occasions you consciously control your breathing by taking a deep breath or by trying to breathe more slowly if you are overly excited. Yet for the most part, you normally breathe in and out over thirty thousand times a day, usually without even giving it a second thought.

The primary function of your lungs is to draw oxygen from the air and pass it on to the bloodstream. This nourishes the blood and every organ of the body. At the same time, the lungs take carbon dioxide (a waste product) from the blood and discharge it back into the air.

THE RESPIRATORY SYSTEM:
STRUCTURE

Your respiratory system is a masterpiece of efficient design. A simple way to describe it is to compare it to an upside-down tree. The main breathing tube (known as the windpipe or *trachea)* is like the tree trunk, which extends from the voice box (called the *pharynx*) into the chest. The windpipe then divides into two branches, known as the *main bronchi,* as seen in Figure 1-1. One goes into the right lung; the other goes into the left. Like two main branches of a tree, each of the two bronchi then divides again and again into smaller bronchi, very much like the larger branches of a tree divide into many tiny branches. These smaller air passages (called *bronchioles*) eventually become microscopic in size, and are approximately ten microns (one one-thousandth millimeter) in diameter. The air passages—both large and small—are surrounded by tiny bands of *smooth muscles,* which are actually wrapped around them. Tiny balloonlike air sacs known as *alveoli* can be found at the end of the bronchioles. When you breathe in, the alveoli expand, and when you breathe out, they contract.

The alveoli are where the main transfer of oxygen and carbon dioxide takes place. Only one one-hundredth inch in diameter when expanded, the alveoli are separated from each other by a thin membrane from the blood vessels of the lung. Oxygen from fresh air is absorbed across this membrane from the lung, while carbon dioxide from the blood passes into the alveoli, to be exhaled through the air passages when we breathe out. The lungs contain over three hundred million tiny alveoli, which cover a total surface area of about eighty square yards —about the size of a regulation tennis court.

The respiratory center in the brain sends messages through the body's autonomic nervous system to maintain the correct intake of air throughout the day and night. It automatically monitors how much oxygen and carbon dioxide are in the blood and determines what our oxygen requirements are at any given moment. When you run to catch a train or climb a flight of stairs, the respiratory center directs the lungs to take in more air to provide the extra oxygen the heart needs to circulate more blood throughout the body. The action is invol-

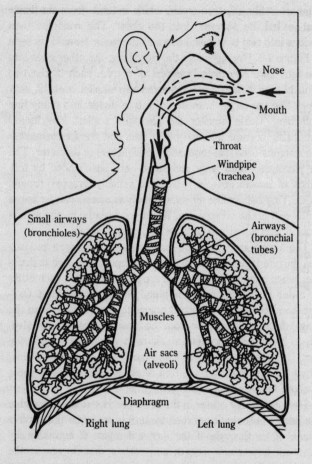

Figure 1-1. The respiratory system, normal lungs. From Thomas F. Plaut, *Children with Asthma: A Manual for Parents*, copyright 1988, Pedipress, Inc. Used with permission.

untary: The muscles do their work without our even thinking about it.

THE RESPIRATORY SYSTEM: OPERATION

When you breathe normally, you inhale air through the nose toward the trachea and lungs, as seen in Figure 1-2. After it enters the nose, the air becomes compressed and is thrown against *mucus,* a sticky coating that lines the nasal passages. Mucus is important, since it traps most of the germs, dust, and other impurities you breathe in. The nasal passages also contain millions of tiny wavy hairs called *cilia,* which are designed to remove old mucus along with the germs, pollen, and dust. Through the cooperative action of the mucus and the cilia, over 95 percent of the dust, pollen, germs, and other impurities you breathe in are removed before the air leaves the nasal passages and proceeds on its way to the lungs.

The nasal passages are not the only place where mucus and cilia exist; they are also found throughout the air passages. When you breathe in minute dust particles or germs through the mouth, the cilia within the air passages send the mucus and impurities back up toward the mouth to be coughed up, spat out, or swallowed. When you swallow germ-laden mucus, it winds up in a sterilizing bath of acid digestive juices in the stomach, to be eliminated later from the body. Though not exactly dinner table conversation, this amazing biological process helps keep the body healthy and free of toxins.

THE ASTHMA FLARE

When you breathe in smoke, fumes, or dust, the mucus traps the impurities. You then are likely to cough, clear your throat,

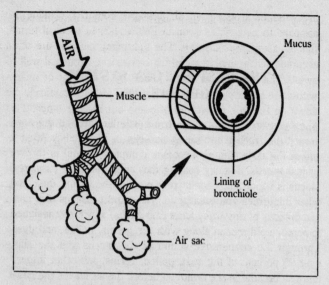

Figure 1-2. Normal bronchiole. Exterior view shows
muscle encircling bronchiole. Cross section shows
normal thickness of muscle, bronchiole lining, and
mucus. From Thomas F. Plaut, *Children with Asthma:
A Manual For Parents,* copyright 1988, Pedipress, Inc.
Used with permission.

and bring up the mucus or phlegm. However, if you have
asthma, you're probably supersensitive to even tiny amounts
of pollen, smoke, dust, and other airborne particles that would
not affect most other people. Doctors describe your airways as
"hyperreactive" or "twitchy," which means that they react in
an exaggerated way to certain stimuli.

During an asthma flare, your bronchi and bronchioles become extremely irritated. To stop the perceived invaders from
entering your lungs, the millions of tiny muscular bands that

are wrapped around your air passages constrict, causing the airspace to narrow, as seen in Figure 1-3. In medical terms, this is called *bronchospasm*. The tightening muscles are often accompanied by irritation, which causes the bronchial wall to swell. This swelling is often joined by a buildup of mucus within the air passage itself. These three factors drastically cut down on the free flow of air into and out of your lungs. This not only prevents the lungs from effectively bringing oxygen into the bloodstream, but also makes it harder for them to remove carbon dioxide from the blood.

Because you have to breathe more deeply and vigorously to maintain an adequate air supply during an asthma episode, the tension within the bronchial walls can increase. This can make your chest feel even tighter and make breathing even more difficult. As a result, both irritation and a buildup of mucus tend to increase in the airways, making an already serious problem even worse. Many asthma patients describe their wheezing and shortness of breath like "breathing through a straw."

At times, your asthma symptoms will subside on their own. However, the vast majority of asthma patients use one or more medications that are designed to open up the air passages. They are known as *bronchodilators* and are taken mostly in aerosol form through the mouth. We'll look into these and other asthma medications in Chapter 6.

IS ASTHMA FATAL?

An asthma attack can be very frightening but is rarely fatal. Even severe attacks can be reversed through proper asthma medications and other medical treatment. Most asthma deaths have been the result of the patient (and the family) being unaware of the severity of the attack until it is too late. Few fatal attacks are sudden, and they often follow several hours or

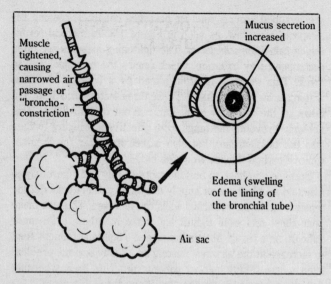

Figure 1-3. Bronchiole during asthma flare. Exterior view shows narrowed bronchioles and overinflated alveoli. Cross section shows narrowed bronchiole almost blocked by swollen lining and increased mucus. From Thomas F. Plaut, *Children with Asthma: A Manual for Parents,* copyright 1988, Pedipress, Inc. Used with permission.

days of the asthma getting worse. This is why both you and your physician need to devise an emergency plan so that you can prevent a severe attack. You should also learn the warning signs that indicate that a severe asthma flare may be developing.

ASTHMA, BRONCHITIS, AND EMPHYSEMA

Some patients wonder if asthma will lead to other lung diseases, such as chronic bronchitis and emphysema. If you are one of these people, take heart! Unless your asthma has been severe or poorly controlled for long periods of time, it will do no permanent damage to your lungs. Chronic bronchitis, which is primarily caused by heavy smoking, involves irritation of the air passages and the production of mucus. Although there is no direct association between the two diseases, many people with bronchitis also suffer from asthma, and certain asthma medications are able to reduce symptoms of bronchitis.

Like chronic bronchitis, emphysema is due to heavy smoking. Asthma does not necessarily lead to emphysema, although smokers with asthma have a much greater risk of coming down with the disease than do nonsmoking asthma patients.

While asthma primarily affects the air passages or bronchioles, emphysema attacks the tiny air sacs of the lungs (the alveoli) and makes them less resilient. This impairs the vital exchange of oxygen and carbon dioxide into the blood and causes a buildup of waste products in the body. Unlike asthma symptoms, which are reversible, the damage to the air sacs is permanent.

For these reasons, smoking cigarettes is especially dangerous to your health if you are suffering from asthma. In addition, secondhand smoke can be harmful to the well-being of members of your household who are suffering from the disease.

Now that we have a basic grounding in what asthma is (and what it is not), let us examine the various factors that can trigger an asthma attack and what you can do to limit your exposure to them.

Please remember that despite the physical and emotional

difficulties involved in having asthma, the prognosis for most asthma patients is good. Through expert diagnosis, aggressive treatment, and conscientious self-care, the vast majority of asthma patients can enjoy all the things that make life worth living: health, travel, work, recreation, exercise, lovemaking, and food. In Part II of this book we offer a comprehensive self-care program that deals with all of these issues.

T W O

WHAT TRIGGERS
ASTHMA?

If you suffer from asthma or know someone who does, you know that a variety of factors can trigger or set off an asthma attack. Many triggers are present in the external environment, and some involve an allergic response. Pollen, dust, animal danders, smoke, fumes, and cold air are among the more common *external* trigger factors that can be breathed in. Certain foods—such as nuts, fish, shellfish, eggs, and milk—and foods containing sulfites are common external asthma triggers that you eat and drink. *Internal* triggers include mechanical factors such as hyperventilation and laughter, as well as exercise and viral infections. In some very sensitive people, even normal body functions such as menstruation and sleeping can set off an asthma flare. Although we will present a long list of asthma trigger factors later on, it is important to remember that the vast majority of asthma sufferers respond to only one or two of them.

Before we explore trigger factors in more detail, let's examine the mechanism in our bodies that opens the door to an asthma attack in certain people. Later we'll provide practical advice on how to avoid and/or control trigger factors.

ALLERGIES

Many experts believe that allergy is a primary component in asthma.

An allergy is simply an overreaction of the immune system (whether minor, such as sneezing or a runny nose, or severe, such as tissue swelling and bronchospasm) to a particular substance that causes no problems in nonallergic individuals. Because of a genetic or other predisposing factor, the immune system of allergy-prone individuals mistakenly identifies a harmless substance entering the body as a threat to health. Allergic reactions primarily affect the skin, the respiratory system, and the blood vessels.

The primary function of the immune system is to protect our body from harmful substances. When it identifies a harmful substance, the immune system attacks the invader (known as an antigen) by producing special white blood cells and special molecules in the blood known as antibodies. But the immune system cannot be activated without having previously met the antigen and identified it as an enemy. Mast cells, a type of white blood cell found in the nose, air passages, and skin, help in this identification process and play a central role in the allergic response among asthma sufferers.

For some reason not fully understood by medical science, the immune system of allergy-prone individuals produces abnormally large numbers of an antibody called IgE (immunoglobin type E). When an antigen such as pollen or dust is breathed into the lungs for the first time, the IgE antibody locks into an appropriate receptor on the mast cell.

Although you may not experience symptoms at the time of your first exposure to an allergen, your mast cell is now sensitized to it: it is primed to respond when you breathe the allergen into the lungs a second time. For example, if you are allergic to ragweed, the "ragweed allergen" was attracted to

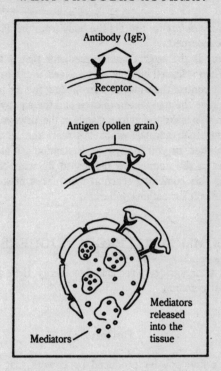

Figure 2-1. The mast cell with antibodies.

the appropriate IgE antibody that was attached to the mast cell the very first time you breathed ragweed pollen into your lungs.

When a second exposure to ragweed takes place, be it hours, days, or weeks later, the antigen forms a bridge across two IgE antibodies that adhere to the mast cell, as seen in Figure 2-1. When this occurs, a type of circuit is closed. The mast cell is then directed to release its store of chemicals (known as *mediators*) to protect the body from the allergen or allergens concerned.

Histamine is the most common mediator that is linked to asthma. When released into the air passages, it can irritate the nerves that control the muscles surrounding the air passages. This can cause the muscles to thicken and the airways to narrow. It can also make the mucus glands in the airways produce more mucus than normal, which obstructs the airways and makes it harder for you to breathe. Histamine can also cause blood cells in the connective tissues to fill with blood and swell. It is this combined reaction that makes breathing extremely difficult for asthma sufferers.

COMMON ALLERGIC TRIGGERS

Dozens of asthma triggers are linked to allergy. Here are some of the most common.

Pollen

Pollen is a fine powder produced by flowers that fertilizes other flowers of the same species so they produce seeds. It is found primarily in the spring and early summer. Ragweed is the most common (and troublesome) source of pollen in the United States and is dreaded by both asthma and hay fever sufferers alike.

Molds

If you feel wheezy during humid weather or when you are exposed to freshly cut grass, chances are that you are allergic to molds. Molds belong to the fungus family and produce a pollenlike dust consisting of millions of spores (a spore is a small cell that enables the fungus to reproduce itself). Molds are most commonly found in warm, damp places and closed spaces. They flourish in damp basements, old wallpaper, upholstery, heavy curtains, thick carpets, humid closets, and damp sheets and pillowcases. Molds can also grow in vaporizers, air conditioners, and humidifiers.

Dust

Most of us think that dust comes only from the outdoors, but it is linked to indoor sources as well. Dust comes from the dead skin cells of humans (dandruff is the most obvious form), fragments of clothing, microscopic debris from upholstery, dead plant matter, and food fragments. It is especially found in animal "dander." Animal dander is made from scales lost from the skin of household pets, especially cats and dogs.

It is not just tiny particles of house dust that can trigger asthma, but also the *house dust mite,* which feeds on dust. Because these microscopic mites can number up to eighteen hundred per gram of dust, most of us never know about their existence, let alone realize that they share our house or apartment with us. Mites live primarily off dead human skin scales and molds. Their favorite places to live include carpets, mattresses, feather pillows, and stuffed toys. Mite feces—which are tiny and light enough to become airborne—can enter the air passages and cause an asthma attack.

Occupational Allergens

This group of specific asthma-related substances are found primarily in the workplace. These are many and varied but are found mostly in the chemical, electronic, and pharmaceutical industries. Because the use of irritants and chemicals in the workplace is increasing all the time, the number of allergens is increasing as well. And because up to several dozen different allergens may be present in the work environment at one time, tracking down such asthma triggers in the workplace is far from easy. Tolulene diisocyanate (TDI), found in the manufacture of polyurethane foam; dander, droppings, urine, and saliva from farm, domestic, and laboratory animals; epoxy resin curing agents used in paint manufacture; wood dusts in the building trades; dusts arising from the cultivation, harvesting, drying, handling, and milling of grains; plant fungi and molds in agribusiness; and allergic reactions to antibiotics, insecticides, and cimetidine in the drug industry are among the most common.

Air Pollutants

Air pollutants can be powerful triggers for asthma attack. In addition to increasing airway reactivity, they can cause the airways to constrict while they increase mucus production. There are three major air pollutants. Sulfur dioxide is caused by the combustion of fossil fuels such as oil and coal. It is a major component in motor vehicle exhaust. Sulfur dioxide triggers bronchoconstriction. Ozone is a component of photochemical smog and causes increased airway reactivity in addition to bronchoconstriction. Nitrogen dioxide is caused by burning. Smokestack discharges from factories is a primary source, although it is caused by gas stoves in the home as well. Nitrogen dioxide is also a major component of cigarette smoke. Like ozone, nitrogen dioxide causes airways to constrict and become hyperreactive. These three major forms of pollution are cited by physicians as a major reason for the increase in asthma in recent years.

Foods

Foods—whether eaten, drunk or inhaled (such as flour dust or vapors given off while food is cooking)—are less common sources of allergy-related asthma, especially among adults. Although there is some controversy about whether specific foods can bring about an asthma attack, the most common problem foods associated with asthma are eggs, cow's milk, shellfish, nuts, wheat, and corn.

NONALLERGENIC TRIGGERS

Some asthma triggers are not related directly to allergy in the strict sense. Doctors refer to these reactions as *idiosyncratic,* because they involve an intolerance to a particular food, drug, or other substance due to an unusual sensitivity. It does not involve a classic immune system response. For example, when we get a runny nose or teary eyes when we're exposed to an irritant such as cigarette smoke, we have an idiosyncratic response to it rather than an allergy. While some asthma-prone people may experience asthma symptoms when exposed to cigarette smoke, the IgE mechanism that defines a true allergic response is not involved.

Food Additives

Medical researchers have focused primarily on several food additives found in a growing number of processed and ready-to-eat foods as nonallergenic asthma triggers.

Tartrazine

Some people become wheezy after eating food colored by tartrazine (yellow food dye no. 5). Tartrazine is found in some brands of cake mixes, soft drinks, and candy. Ironically, it can even be found in certain medications, including some used to treat asthma.

Sulfites

Sulfites are chemicals routinely added to many foods to preserve color and give an appearance of freshness. Sulfites are listed under a wide variety of names, including sulfur dioxide, sodium and potassium bisulfite, sodium and potassium metabisulfite, and sodium sulfite. In addition to being added to certain raw vegetables in salad bars in delicatessens and restaurants, sulfites are often found in fruit drinks, most brands of beer and wine, baked goods, seafood products (especially shrimp), dried fruit, and many processed foods. Until food providers remove all sulfites from foods, we consumers are mostly on our own. Be sure to check the product label or ask your waiter in the restaurant if sulfites are used. Many over-the-counter and prescribed medications—including some to treat asthma—contain sulfites. Since it is unlikely that you'll be told whether the medication you need contains sulfites, check with your pharmacist to make sure.

Molds

Foods that naturally contain molds include mushrooms, most types of cheeses, sour cream and buttermilk, wine and beer breads (such as pumpernickel and sourdough) that are made with lots of yeast, smoked and pickled foods such as sauer kraut and sausages, dried fruits, products containing vinegar (such as mayonnaise, ketchup, and pickles), and just about any meat that has been left standing for more than a day or two.

Beta Blockers

These drugs are routinely used to treat heart disease and high blood pressure and can trigger asthma.

Aspirin

Aspirin and products containing aspirin sometimes trigger asthma attack in sensitive individuals. Although severe (and sudden) attacks are rare, studies show that at least one asthma patient in ten experiences a drop in lung function of 20 percent after taking aspirin. Most popular brands include Bayer, Alka-Seltzer, Bufferin, Ecotrin, and aspirin formula Excedrin, Vanquish, Midol, and Anacin.

Ibuprofen

Certain aspirin-free drugs known as "nonsteroidal and anti-inflammatory medications" that treat symptoms of pain, headache, arthritis and menstrual cramps can produce asthma symptoms in aspirin-sensitive individuals. The most popular of these, such as Motrin, Advil, and Nuprin, contain ibuprofen. For this reason, sensitive individuals are advised to take drugs containing acetaminophen (such as Tylenol) instead.

Infections

Infections can be caused by viruses (such as the common cold or flu), bacteria (including strep throat and pneumonia), and molds. Viral infections in the respiratory tract can damage the respiratory lining and increase bronchial sensitivity. For this reason, viruses involving the nose, throat, and bronchial tubes tend to provoke most asthma attacks due to infection.

Gastrointestinal Reflux

This involves the regurgitation of digestive fluid through the opening between the stomach and the esophagus. For most people this only produces a case of heartburn, but for asthma-prone individuals it can precipitate an asthma attack or severe coughing. Reflux often occurs at night during sleep.

Exercise

When we exercise, our lungs work more quickly and exchange air more rapidly than when we are lying down, walking, or standing still. Because the nose is unable to condition this air as it does under normal circumstances, the untreated (and often cold) air goes directly into the trachea and lungs. The air passages tend to dry out and lose the moist blanket of mucus that normally protects them. As a result, the air passages become very sensitive. In asthma-prone individuals the mast cells in the respiratory tract begin to release mediators so that inflammation of the air passages occurs in a way similar to their response to an allergen. An asthma attack can be the result.

This does not mean that asthma-prone individuals should

give up exercise. In fact, exercise is recommended for people with asthma. As we see in Chapter 10, people with exercise-induced asthma need to learn how to adjust their exercise so it can be tolerated. In addition, they can select those forms of exercise (such as swimming) that are less likely to trigger an attack in the first place.

Emotions

Anger, depression, fear, and sadness are believed to trigger asthma flares in certain individuals. One prevailing theory teaches that emotions such as anger, fear, and depression can trigger asthma directly. Although there is no hard medical evidence to support this belief, it has been well established in medical literature that thoughts, attitudes, and emotions can affect our immune response.

As far as asthma and allergy are concerned, attention has focused on the number of *eosinophils,* which are white blood cells that are often found in the blood during allergic reactions. Studies have established that feelings of helplessness or "giving up" can increase the number of eosinophils in the blood, while feelings of self-sufficiency can reduce them.

Mechanical Events

Another prevailing belief is that emotions can trigger asthma attacks indirectly, through *mechanical events.* If a child is angry at her mother, she may yell and stomp out of the room. The yelling upsets the normal breathing pattern and can trigger an asthma attack. Because the same response would occur if the child were acting out the role of being angry and yelled at her mother in a school play, allergists point out that it isn't the emotion but the mechanical event that triggers asthma. Most of us know that when we are angry, sad, or experience feelings of mirth or delight, our breathing rate increases. This change in breathing may cause you to hyperventilate, which can trigger an asthma flare. Many asthma patients I have interviewed often have difficulty distinguishing between the emotional state and the mechanical event before experiencing an asthma flare, so it seems that it hardly matters which of these two theories is correct. There would appear to be some truth in both, although there is still some disagreement among asthma specialists regarding these distinctions.

In Part II we explore how we can track down individual asthma triggers, and we find out how they can be dealt with.

THREE

IF YOUR CHILD
HAS ASTHMA

If you have a child with asthma, you know how difficult life can be. In this chapter we offer ideas about how life with asthma can be easier for you, your child, and the rest of the family.

Approximately one child in ten will experience asthma symptoms at some time in his or her life. As the most common chronic illness in childhood, asthma is the leading cause of absenteeism from school, and it causes more hospital visits (including some 150,000 emergency room admissions) than any other childhood disease.

Asthma often appears for the first time between two and five years of age, and it appears to be twice as common among boys as among girls. Children who have been breast-fed from birth tend to be less sensitive to trigger factors of asthma than children who were fed on bottled formula. According to medical statistics, two thirds of all asthmatic children basically outgrow asthma by their midteens, although some of them occasionally experience symptoms as adults. Although most asthma attacks are mild, some can be very severe indeed.

We include a separate chapter on asthma and children because asthma affects children differently than adults. Asthma in a child affects physical growth, school attendance, and participation in sports and play, and children with asthma often need to deal with feeling "different" more than most other children do. Feelings of inferiority, guilt, anger, and depression are common psychological traits among children with asthma.

These problems do not affect only the children; asthma also has a powerful impact on the entire family. Asthma attacks can be terrifying experiences, both for the child and other family members. In addition to placing an additional financial burden on the family, children with asthma (especially when they are young) often require constant attention and monitoring by the mother and father. Parents may be reluctant to leave their asthmatic child with a baby-sitter and or hesitant to let them spend the day or night with their friends. When a child in the family has asthma, discipline is often a problem. Many parents try not to upset the child and possibly trigger an asthma attack. Needless to say, all of these special concerns place tremendous stress on the family.

One of the most damaging myths parents and children believe about childhood asthma is that "there really isn't much I can do" to manage asthma symptoms. Far too many parents place responsibility for care on the physician, and wait until a serious flare-up of symptoms appears before they take corrective action. This attitude is not only dangerous to the child's health, it also can bring about deep psychological trauma for all concerned.

According to Dr. David A. Mrazek of the National Jewish Center for Immunology and Respiratory Medicine, approximately 90 percent of all children affected by asthma have the potential to lead a "very full life." Nine percent will be limited in some way by their disease, while asthma is "crippling" for only 1 percent. Like adults, the vast majority of children with asthma, and their parents, can effectively manage asthma at home.

By understanding the basic physical, psychological, and social issues involved in childhood asthma we can become better educated about the disease and how it affects the child and the family. While this groundwork will be laid in this chapter, specific information regarding the diagnosis and management of childhood asthma will be included, where appropriate, in following chapters.

ASTHMA SYMPTOMS IN CHILDREN

How do you know that your child has asthma? For the most part, the symptoms of asthma in children are similar to those of adults. However, since the child's respiratory system is smaller and the air passages narrower than those of older people, symptoms often take place faster and occur with less warning. According to Thomas F. Plaut, M.D., in his excellent book *Children with Asthma,* there are in children four signs of asthma trouble that parents should watch for:

1. **Wheezing.** This high-pitched sound occurs when the air passages narrow during an asthma attack. It usually begins only when the child breathes out, but it can become progressively louder if the attack becomes more severe. In a moderate to severe attack, wheezing can also be heard when the child inhales.

2. **Chest skin is sucked in.** During an asthma attack, the skin between the ribs appears to be sucked in. This happens because air cannot be drawn into the lungs fast enough.

3. **Breathing out takes longer than breathing in.** During a moderate attack it may take up to twice as long to exhale as to inhale.

4. **Increased breathing rate.** During a moderate attack, the child's breathing rate can increase to 50 percent above nor-

mal. If the breathing rate increases beyond this point, the attack is considered to be severe.

The first asthma episode—especially if moderate or severe —can be terrifying experience for both you and your child. While some attacks will subside by themselves, the first episode usually requires the care of a qualified physician. For many parents this will involve the child's pediatrician. Bring your child to your physician for a thorough examination and appropriate treatment without delay, because untreated asthma symptoms tend to get worse rather than improve. By being aware of the four warning signs, you as a parent can summon help before the asthma flare reaches a crisis stage requiring a visit to a hospital emergency room.

CHILDHOOD TRIGGER FACTORS AND THEIR CONTROL

Many of the trigger factors described in the previous chapter are equally irritating to children and to adults, including allergy, cold air, smoke and other irritants, exercise, and food. However, the predominant trigger factors for children appear to involve viral respiratory infections such as colds, as well as allergens. Mechanical events, which include laughing, crying, or yelling, are also common. Most children with asthma may be affected by only one or two trigger factors, while a tiny minority will be adversely affected by most or all of them.

Several new studies of childhood asthma have suggested that the family environment plays a major role in successful asthma management. Children from chaotic and unstable family environments tend to have more asthma flares, while children from predictable and stable family environments have less.

As we've pointed out earlier, asthma, especially if it is

chronic or prolonged, can have a profound effect on both the patient and the family. For many children with asthma, their lives are literally *shaped* by their illness, which often affects their relationships with family and friends as well as their self-image, life goals, future career, and even marriage possibilities.

THE PHYSICAL IMPACT OF ASTHMA

If your child has asthma, you are probably dealing with at least some of the following physical issues involving exercise.

Breathing during an asthma attack is more difficult than it is under normal conditions. As a result, a child with asthma has to work much harder to maintain an adequate intake of oxygen than other children do. When asthma is chronic, the child's heart, lungs, and chest muscles are almost always working overtime. This makes the child often feel tired and run-down.

In addition, children whose asthma is triggered by exercise tend to restrict physical activity in order to prevent an attack. They avoid taking gym classes, and they choose not to participate in organized sports and other physically taxing group activities. This often begins a vicious circle. As a result of restricting their physical activity, children with asthma are often out of shape. This makes physical activity more of an effort, so they do less and less. An estimated 80 percent of the children admitted to the National Jewish Center for Immunology and Respiratory Medicine—which sees patients with more serious and uncontrolled asthma—do not participate in physical education programs at their home or school. Through the Center's unique program of evaluation, asthma education, and exercise, nearly all patients can take gym classes by the time they are discharged.

Doctors and physical therapists stress that regular exercise is essential for asthma patients of all ages and that parents should not restrict their child's activity just because he or she has asthma. By choosing the best exercises, pacing themselves, and taking preventive medications when necessary, most children with asthma can participate fully in nearly every kind of physical activity both in and out of school. This not only makes them more physically fit, it also helps them feel better about themselves. In Chapter 10 we examine the best types of exercise for people with asthma.

SEVERE, CHRONIC ASTHMA

If your child suffers from severe, chronic, or poorly controlled asthma, the following issues are of special importance to both you and your child.

Growth

Although mild to moderate asthma does not usually retard normal growth patterns, asthma that is severe, chronic, or poorly controlled can retard the normal growth of children. In addition, prolonged use of steroids to control asthma can interfere with the normal growth of certain patients.

Posture

When a child has severe asthma, the shoulder and neck muscles tend to be used for breathing in addition to the chest muscles alone. In chronic cases the child tends to hold the shoulders high and forward. After several years this can give the child a round-shouldered posture with a concave, pulled-in chest. In addition, prolonged use of steroids to control asthma can stimulate appetite, which leads to weight gain. This is responsible for the round-faced look found among some young asthma patients.

ASTHMA: RARELY FATAL

Even though we've said it before, it is important to remember that asthma is rarely fatal. Only 1 percent of all children with asthma have extremely severe and chronic asthma, and among them only a small percentage can die from an asthma attack. However, for the vast majority of young patients whose asthma is not severe and can be controlled with low order medications, the chances of dying from asthma are remote indeed. According to Emlen H. Jones, M.D., writing in *Children with Asthma,* only one of twenty-five thousand children with asthma will die during a given year.

MANAGING SYMPTOMS

As we pointed out earlier, asthma symptoms are reversible and do not by themselves lead to emphysema or permanent lung damage such as scarring. For the most part permanent heart damage does not occur either, except in very severe cases where asthma is chronic and out of control. This is one reason why doctors stress the importance of aggressive management when severe asthma is present.

THE PSYCHOLOGICAL IMPACT
OF ASTHMA

Because all children are different, asthma will affect them (as well as their families) in different ways. Much depends on the severity of the asthma, how well it is controlled, and whether a strong support system exists for both the child and the family.

This especially holds true from a psychological standpoint. Psychologists point out that there is no one "asthma personality." Children with asthma exhibit the same range of emotions as children who are asthma-free. However, like other children with a chronic disease, young asthma sufferers often experience a range of emotions particular to them.

Anger and Resentment

These two emotions are common among children with asthma, especially if the disease is chronic or poorly controlled. They feel betrayed by their own bodies and often feel victimized and resentful. These feelings may be acted out directly or in more subtle ways. For example, some children express anger directly through sarcasm, cruelty, or temper tantrums. Others may express anger covertly by manipulating others or by making others feel sorry for them.

Fear

For many young patients, a trip to a hospital emergency room can be more traumatic than the attack itself. Because most children are neither aware how an asthma flare comes about nor what can be done to prevent it, they may feel both resigned to and terrified about the next attack. Although many children don't speak about it, there is also a fear of death or permanent disability, especially if the asthma is severe. For this reason, doctors stress the importance of education and psychological support for young asthma patients. This team effort has two practical aspects. First, it has been found that when the patient, the parents, and the physician work together to understand and manage asthma, its triggers, and its symptoms, the disease can be more effectively controlled through medication and other means. Second, the child feels a greater sense of control and empowerment over his or her condition. This increases as the child becomes proficient at monitoring the condition. As a result there is less fear, both on the part of the child *and* the parents.

Inferiority Feelings

Because children with chronic, poorly controlled asthma are often unable to compete physically with other children, they feel that they don't measure up. This not only makes them want to avoid physical activities such as sports and other active games, it also can hurt their social life as well.

Guilt and Depression

Like feelings of inferiority, guilt and depression are especially intense among children with chronic or severe asthma. They often feel that they are a burden on their family and friends, especially in the aftermath of a severe asthma flare. The perception of being inferior and different can lead to feelings of worthlessness. Some of the medications used to treat asthma, such as oral steroids, can bring about feelings of depression as well. Asthma patients who are steroid-dependent are more

likely to become clinically depressed. Symptoms include prolonged mood changes involving sadness, hopelessness, irrita-
bility, and listlessness. Depression may also involve changes in
eating and sleeping habits and marked changes in schoolwork
and friendships. Depression among young asthma patients is a
worrisome sign, because those (especially teens) who are
chronically depressed tend to ignore the warnings of a serious
attack or may choose not to take their medication properly.
In fact, depression is now being considered as a major factor
in the gradual rise of asthma fatalities among young people
today.

STRATEGIES FOR PARENTS
AND CHILDREN: A TEAM EFFORT

Here are a number of ways in which you and your child can
take charge of the situation:

Education

If your child has asthma, it is absolutely essential that you
learn everything possible about the disease in general and how
it affects your child in particular. In short, you need to know
the facts. This involves reading books, speaking to the family
doctor or asthma specialist, and seeking information from
asthma organizations and parent support groups. A listing of
major groups can be found in the Asthma Sources section at
the back of this book. The previously mentioned *Children with
Asthma* should be read by every parent of a child with asthma.
It is often available through your doctor's office or it can be

obtained from the address given in the Recommended Reading section.

Gaining knowledge about asthma should not be limited to you as a parent. Children are naturally curious, and they want to know what they can do to help themselves. Even young children are able to understand the basics of their disease and what can trigger asthma symptoms. As your child gets older, he or she can learn much about the mechanics of bronchospasm, its causes, and how to manage its symptoms. By the time your child is a teenager, he or she should become an expert in the understanding and management of the disease.

Home Care

One of the major aspects of effective asthma management is teaching both you and your child how to handle attacks at home. Learning how to know when an attack may be imminent, how to measure lung capacity through the use of a peak flow meter, how to choose and administer the proper medications with the metered dose inhaler or nebulizer, how to make sure that your child is taking medications regularly and in the proper dosage, and when to seek professional help when an attack becomes dangerous are some of the goals of parent-child education.

Many parents give their doctor primary responsibility for relieving asthma symptoms. This creates undue dependency on the physician; in addition, unexpected symptoms can sometimes get so serious that you need to take your child to a hospital emergency room for treatment. This can often be very traumatic for both you and your child. For this reason, you, your child, and your physician must learn to work together as a team to develop effective home strategies to deal with often unexpected asthma flares.

School

For many young asthma patients, school presents a number of challenges they do not have to deal with at home. Feeling excluded from certain school activities is upsetting to some children because they feel isolated from other classmates. However, the young patient's major problem is how to deal with an asthma flare while at school. For this reason, effective asthma management at school can limit the disruptive effects of an asthma attack, both for the child and for others in school.

Like the strategies for effective home care presented earlier, a team approach at school is needed. After your child's asthma is diagnosed and evaluated by the physician, you, the teachers, the school nurse, and the school counselor need to develop a strategy to help meet your child's needs. First there must be a clear understanding of what your child can do and what he or she cannot do in school, when the child needs to take medication, and when you should be called in an emergency. Draw up specific plans of action in the event of an asthma flare. The role of the teacher or other responsible person at school should be clearly defined. For example, the following four-step plan has been outlined by a parent for her eight-year-old boy we'll call Kevin:

1. If Kevin begins wheezing or feels tightness in his chest have him sit down; relax; and take deep, regular breaths This may help him relax and get his breathing under control.

2. If Kevin is upset, perhaps offer a glass of warm water as a diversionary tactic to get him to think of something else.

3. Help him find his metered dose inhaler (it is held for safe keeping at the principal's office). The doctor suggests that he take two whiffs with at least a two-minute interval between the first and the second dose.

4. If symptoms do not subside, please call me at my office number.

In addition to your contact number at home or at work, the telephone number of the child's physician should also be noted in the event that you cannot be reached. By drawing up a plan beforehand, much confusion can be avoided if an asthma flare at school occurs.

It is also important that you as a parent stay in touch with the school staff to make certain that these preventive strategies can actually work. For example, you might call the teacher to inform him or her about your child's health status on a particular day. When it comes to effective asthma management at school, you are usually called on to take primary responsibility for reaching out to faculty and counselors and creating a working team. Very often it is the parent who needs to provide to the school staff accurate information about asthma and how to manage it.

Summer Camp

Finally, summer camps for children can be very effective in providing them with asthma education, coping skills, emotional support, and exercise. They are also a lot of fun and provide new friendships and peer models. As a result, summers in asthma camp can help your child to become more knowledgeable about the disease and to build self-confidence and self-reliance.

THE SUPPORT SYSTEM FOR PARENTS

Being a parent is difficult even under the best of circumstances. However, parenting a child with a chronic disease such as asthma can be one of the most demanding challenges you will ever have. Although many of us try to be supermoms and superdads, coping with asthma in the family may become too large a burden to handle alone. For this reason, emotional support is often recommended. What kind of support system are we talking about?

One-to-One

For some parents, a support system can include a number of trusted friends, relatives, or clergy. For others it may include the family doctor or asthma specialist. You may need to seek the help of a social worker or psychotherapist who has experience with chronic diseases.

Groups

In many communities there are special support groups for parents of children with asthma. Some may be part of a group such as Mothers of Asthmatics (see Asthma Sources in the back of this book) or affiliated with a local medical center, mental health association, or lung association. Support groups may be free, or on an ability-to-pay basis. In addition, there are a growing number of support groups specifically for children with asthma. Call the National Jewish Center for Immunology and Respiratory Medicine's toll-free "LUNG-LINE" at 800-222-LUNG (303-388-4461 in Colorado) to find out about the location of an asthma support group near you.

The key to successful asthma management is not to let the disease take control of your life, and to learn how to work creatively with the challenges it brings. By learning about the disease itself; identifying early warning signs; recognizing trig ger factors; understanding the lab tests, management procedures, and medications; and learning good health and exercise habits, both you and your child can do much to prevent and control childhood asthma symptoms. By taking an active role, you and your family become empowered. You respect the disease but are not defeated by it. This feeling of empowerment creates benign cycles within the family that can enhance self-esteem and mutual caring and can lead to closer and more harmonious relationships.

FOUR

ASTHMA AND PREGNANCY

Many women with asthma are worried about the consequences of getting pregnant. They wonder whether pregnancy will make their asthma worse, or if having an asthma attack can cause harm to their baby. They are especially worried that a major decrease in their breathing during a severe attack will deprive their baby of needed oxygen and cause death or mental retardation. Others ask if any special precautions must be taken to improve their chances of having an easy pregnancy and normal delivery. These are important concerns, but if you are a woman with asthma who is planning to have a baby, the news is good.

Studies in the United States and Europe have shown that for the vast majority of women, asthma will not complicate pregnancy or childbirth in any way. In fact, asthma complications (such as oxygen deprivation, stillbirths, and infant deaths) affect only 1 percent of all pregnancies, and these are primarily among women with the most severe, debilitating asthma symptoms that are not controlled. If proper medical care is taken both during pregnancy and after the baby's birth, the risk of problems are minimized. On the following pages we briefly discuss the special questions and needs of the prospective mother with asthma.

WILL ASTHMA MAKE PREGNANCY MORE DIFFICULT?

Studies have shown that for about half the pregnant women with asthma, pregnancy will not produce any major changes in their asthma condition. Approximately 20 percent experience a worsening of symptoms, while some 30 percent experience a general improvement in their asthma condition. Studies have shown that asthma flares rarely occur during the last four weeks of pregnancy, and attacks during labor are rare. However, some women may experience periods of breathlessness toward the end of their pregnancy. This is not because of asthma but is due to the fact that they have to breathe both for themselves and the new baby. They also have a full womb pressing against their lungs!

If you are a woman with asthma, go for a thorough medical evaluation by an asthma specialist as soon as you learn that you are pregnant. This will not only help decrease your chances of asthma flares, but also you can learn how best to manage them if they occur. In addition to performing a basic physical examination, the doctor will do a variety of pulmonary function tests to determine your lung capacity and peak flow rate. If you have only a vague idea of the factors that trigger your asthma, tests to help identify these triggers may also be done. You then can try to reduce exposure to triggers such as pollen, molds, and animal dander. If exercise is a trigger for asthma, you can take a bronchodilator before exercising.

In general, doctors advise against drinking alcohol for all women during pregnancy, as it can lead to various degrees of growth abnormality, mental retardation, and behavioral problems for the baby. Avoid cigarette smoke if you are pregnant, especially if you suffer from asthma.

WILL ASTHMA DRUGS HARM THE BABY?

Asthma specialists both here and in Europe report that the vast majority of medications used in asthma management cannot affect the embryo or fetus and will not harm the baby in any way. The only drugs that can cause potential harm are oral steroids, but if they are taken in prescribed amounts, danger is minimized. In general, asthma patients should take the minimal amount of medication necessary to control their asthma, and pregnant women are no exception. Always consult with your obstetrician about specific medications you are taking during pregnancy, and how they can affect the health of your baby.

HOW WILL ASTHMA AFFECT LABOR?

For the vast majority of pregnant women, asthma will not have a negative impact on the birthing process. In fact, it has been found that during labor, the adrenal glands pour out large quantities of cortisones and adrenaline into the blood; this minimizes the chances of having an asthma flare.

Nevertheless, it is always good sense for the hospital staff to know that you have asthma before you come into the delivery room. This may help determine what anesthesia (if any) is to be used, especially if an emergency cesarean section may be necessary. It is also good to have your asthma medication handy, just in case it is needed. For women with serious asthma, extra precautions should be taken with the physician beforehand.

WHAT ABOUT BREAST-FEEDING?

Breast-feeding is highly recommended for newborns in general and for children of mothers with asthma in particular. Asthma specialists believe that the chance that the baby will ingest asthma drugs from mother's milk is extremely remote, and asthma has not been found to decrease the production of breast milk in any way. In addition to the general psychological and health benefits breast-feeding can provide for the infant, it is believed actually to help protect babies from developing certain allergic conditions that may trigger asthma symptoms.

However, in rare cases asthma drugs such as steroids or theophylline can be passed from a mother to her baby through breast milk. If you are taking either of these medications, consult with your doctor regarding the benefits of breast-feeding versus any risks that may affect your baby's health. If you are taking theophylline and are breast-feeding your baby, a blood test may be recommended to see if this drug is being passed along to your baby through the milk.

When a woman becomes pregnant, she is likely to experience many physical and emotional changes. The concerns and fears that many women with asthma have about pregnancy are normal. However, by following the guidelines presented in this and later chapters, asthma should pose no special dangers to either you or your baby.

PART II
MANAGING
ASTHMA

FIVE

THE MEDICAL DIAGNOSIS

If you believe that you or a member of your family may be suffering from asthma, a thorough, careful, and objective medical diagnosis is essential. This not only helps you and your doctor decide on the best course of prevention and treatment, it also lets you monitor the effects of the treatment itself, which may need to be changed from time to time. Generally speaking, a proper diagnosis of asthma involves a complete medical history, a thorough physical examination, and a variety of laboratory tests. Let's see what is involved in this important process.

FINDING A PHYSICIAN

If you or a family member has trouble breathing, seeking out a physician is a top priority. But which doctor to choose? Here are a few suggestions.

The Family Doctor

When most people have symptoms of coughing or wheezing, the family doctor is often the first to be consulted. This is usually a good idea, because he or she is most familiar with your health history. The family doctor (who is often a general practitioner or GP) is also likely to be aware of specific personality traits, family situations, and life-style habits that may have a bearing on your health as well. Your family doctor also knows which prescribed medications you are taking and what you may be allergic to.

The General Practitioner

Some general practitioners specialize in asthma. However, many have insufficient training in asthma diagnosis and treatment. As a result, some patients become frustrated because they feel that their asthma is not under control. According to Drs. John L. Decker and Michael A. Kaliner of The National Institutes of Health, you should consider seeking out another doctor if the following are true relative to treatment of asthma:

1. There is no improvement after three to six months of care.

2. You or your child has to visit an emergency room more than once a year.

3. You are using oral steroids daily.

4. Your present physician is unable to provide detailed explanations about your course of treatment.

A good general practitioner will refer you to an asthma doctor, such as a pulmonologist (a lung specialist) or an allergist (a specialist in allergies). However, you shouldn't hesitate to seek out a specialist on your own just because your doctor does not refer you to one.

The Asthma Specialist

If you do not have a family doctor at present or if your asthma symptoms are sudden or severe, you may want to consult an asthma specialist right away. However, not all pulmonologists or allergists are specialists in asthma, so find out beforehand. For the most part, these physicians have far more training and knowledge in diagnosing and treating asthma than most general practitioners do. Since *your* health is at stake, it's always a good idea to get the best care you possibly can.

Residential Treatment

Some patients with very serious and chronic asthma may require a period in a residential treatment program for asthma. One such program at the National Jewish Center for Immunology and Respiratory Medicine lasts two to five weeks and offers a multidisciplinary, comprehensive approach. Primary care includes a complete physical evaluation of the patient, and a medical program to control asthma symptoms. The second stage of the program helps the patient to identify trigger factors and offers instruction on the use of medications, symptom monitoring, dietary advice, exercise instruction, and management strategies. It also includes psychological and social evaluations. This comprehensive approach to asthma management is both highly successful and cost-effective. The results after a three-year follow-up of twenty-nine patients showed a 62 percent reduction in hospitalizations, a 64 percent reduction in hospital days, and a 48 percent reduction in emergency room visits.

TOWARD A GOOD PATIENT-DOCTOR RELATIONSHIP

Whether you are seeing a GP or an asthma specialist, it is important that both you and your physician have a good working relationship based on trust and mutual respect. Asthma often provokes a good deal of stress and frustration in the patient, who understandably wants to get rid of the symptoms as quickly (and as permanently) as possible. Some go to the physician expecting a miracle cure. It is important that both you and your doctor sit down to discuss (1) what the diagnosis involves, (2) what asthma is and what it is not, and (3) what to expect from the course of treatment.

For the most part, the more you know about asthma, the better the chances that you'll have a realistic idea of how it can be managed. In addition, you will have more success in managing your asthma if you take a share of the responsibility for your care, rather than leaving it completely in the hands of your physician.

The best asthma treatment program involves the *whole person* rather than the lungs alone. For this reason you may want to consider a physician who is not only concerned about your pulmonary functions but who is also interested in education, preventive strategies, home care, diet, and exercise. It is also important that you be told about any physical and psychological issues associated with the disease itself (such as possible fatigue or frustration) as well as any adverse reactions you can expect to asthma medications.

For assistance in finding an asthma doctor, call National Jew-

ish's "LUNG-LINE" (see the Asthma Sources section) for a
list of practitioners in your area.

THE FIRST VISIT

When you consult a physician for the first time, you will be
asked to fill out a medical history. A complete, accurate, and
truthful medical history is very important. In addition to building an important foundation for an accurate diagnosis, it lays
the groundwork for future asthma care. A good medical history form will ask questions about your personal and family
health history, your work environment and hobbies, specific
life-style habits (such as smoking), any allergies you already
know about, and factors (such as specific foods or exercise)
that you suspect may trigger symptoms. You will be asked
about the onset, pattern, intensity, and frequency of symptoms, and how these symptoms affect your life both physically
and emotionally. Mention any previous treatment for asthma
and what (if any) medications you may be taking. Do not hesitate to add any additional information you feel may be important for the doctor to know. If you're in doubt, mention it
anyway.

THE PHYSICAL EXAM

The physical examination is also important. It helps the doctor
to get a good overall view of your general physical condition as
well as enabling him or her to arrive at an accurate asthma
diagnosis. In an exam for asthma, special attention will be de-
voted to any signs and symptoms associated with allergy. This
will include an examination of your chest that will most likely
focus on heartbeat and breathing rate. The doctor will also

listen for wheezing, examine the muscles of the diaphragm, and determine if there is mucus present in the airways.

The doctor will also examine your nose and nasal passages to look for signs of sinusitis (inflammation of the sinuses), nasal polyps, or any structural abnormalities of the nasal passages that can have an impact on asthma.

X RAYS

Your physician may recommend a chest X ray to rule out heart disease or other lung problems, such as cystic fibrosis in children, that tend to mimic asthma symptoms. The chest X ray can also reveal conditions of the lung that are associated with asthma, such as pneumonia or the presence of mucus plugs in the airways. If your asthma is severe, the physician may want to take an X ray of the sinuses as well.

In addition to X rays, doctors often order a variety of other laboratory tests. They can be either simple or complex, and tend to vary according to what the physician feels is necessary to achieve a complete and accurate evaluation.

ELECTROCARDIOGRAM

For patients over forty years of age, an electrocardiogram (EKG) is often performed. Its purpose is to help the doctor understand the heart's rhythm and to make sure you aren't suffering from heart failure, a disease that can sometime mimic asthma symptoms.

BLOOD TESTS

A blood test in asthma diagnosis is common, and different types of tests reveal a variety of information. Basically, the blood test reveals the red blood count. If your red blood count is high, it indicates that the level of oxygen in the circulating blood is low. Breathing problems can intensify this problem.

A blood test can indicate whether your asthma symptoms are allergy-related; when asthma is triggered by an allergic response, the number of a particular type of white blood cells called *eosinophils* may increase.

A blood test can also reveal the level of sugar present in your blood. A high blood sugar level can indicate the presence of diabetes. Not only is this a serious disease in itself, but also the presence of diabetes may interfere with the effectiveness of several medications used to treat asthma.

Arterial Gases Test

An arterial gases test evaluates the amount of oxygen and carbon dioxide present in the blood. It is especially useful when taken during a severe asthma flare because it can provide important information about how your lungs function under the stress of an asthma episode.

RAST

A new, more sophisticated blood test that is sometimes used in the diagnosis of asthma is known as RAST (radioallergosorbent test). It measures the amount of chemicals in the immune system that can set off an allergic reaction. Specifically, it measures the quantities of IgE (immunoglobulin type

E) in particular allergens. A high IgE count indicates that asthma due to allery is probably present.

PRIST and ELISA

Other blood tests include the PRIST (paper radioimmunosorbent test), which can measure the total amount of IgE in the blood. The ELISA (enzyme-linked immuno-assay test) has become widely known for its ability detect the HIV (human immunodeficiency virus) antibody in the blood. However, it has also been used for asthma patients because it can, by using an enzyme marker, measure the amount of IgE in specific allergens. These two tests and the RAST test have been considered good alternatives to some of the numerous skin tests that have traditionally been performed on asthma patients to measure their responses to specific allergens. Because the RAST and PRIST tests are both relatively new and sophisticated, they are not yet widely available to asthma patients.

SPUTUM ANALYSIS

Sputum is the substance expelled when you cough or clear your throat. It contains mucus, cellular debris, and a variety of microorganisms. When examined under a microscope, sputum may also contain eosinophils, mold, and mucus plugs, which form in the air passages during an asthma attack. For this reason, a sputum analysis can be helpful in asthma diagnosis.

LUNG FUNCTION TESTS

To make an accurate diagnosis, the doctor needs to know how well your lungs are functioning.

Spirometry

The spirometry test is designed to measure the volume of air that can be expelled from the lungs, as well as the amount of resistance to the flow of air in the respiratory tract when you breathe out. As you breathe into a mouthpiece, the spirometer records the volume of air breathed in and out (as well as the time it takes to do it) on graph paper. The results are then analyzed. Very often this test is given both before and after a bronchodilator (a medicine designed to open up the air passages) is used to determine both the reversability of symptoms and whether you have asthma in the first place. If your pulmonary function is not affected by the bronchodilator, emphysema may be suspected instead of asthma. Spirometry is also used on subsequent visits to the physician to help determine the success of asthma treatment over an extended period of time.

Bronchial Challenge Tests

A variety of bronchial challenge tests may be given when spirometry finds that your air flow and lung volume capacity are normal. Challenge tests often involve introducing "real life" stimuli such as a suspected allergen (for example, pollen), exercise, or cold air. Lung capacity and airflow are then mea-

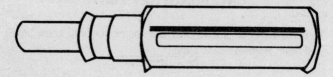

Figure 5-1. The mini-Wright peak-flow meter.

sured. For example, to determine the degree of exercise-induced asthma, the following procedure may take place. First, your lung functions would be measured with a spirometer and a *peak-flow meter*, illustrated in Figure 5-1. You would then be asked to walk or run on a treadmill for a determined length of time. The doctor would measure your pulmonary response ten to fifteen minutes after the exercise, since exercise-induced bronchospasm is often delayed.

Peak-flow meter. Every asthma patient should learn how to measure expiratory flow (the amount of air exhaled) through a peak-flow meter. It is a simple, hand-held device consisting of a tube and an indicator. You blow into the device as fast and as hard as possible, and the figure obtained is a measurement of the flow in liters of air per minute (L/M). The normal peak flow depends on your age, size, and sex; a man who is six feet tall and weighs 180 pounds will have a higher peak flow than a girl of twelve who weighs ninety-five pounds. Your physician can tell you what your normal expiratory flow should be. The best level of peak flow should fall within 20 percent of either side of your predicted normal volume. Measuring your peak-flow rate several times a day can help you predict when a asthma flare is coming on, as well as reveal how your medications are working after a flare has occurred. It also helps you to find out if you were exposed to a trigger factor. Keeping a careful record of peak flow several times daily also helps both you and your physician to adjust medications used to treat asthma.

SKIN TESTING

Because it is often difficult to pinpoint specific allergens through breath tests alone, a variety of skin tests are also used to determine which specific allergens may trigger asthma symptoms. Specifically, a skin test can help confirm that wheeziness is indeed an asthmatic response and is not due to another lung problem. It can also be helpful in prevention and treatment. For example, if you know that you are allergic to cat dander, you can take appropriate medication before visiting the home of a friend who has several cats.

There are basically two types of skin tests used in asthma diagnosis. One test involves scratching the top layers of skin with a needle in different locations (usually on the arm, back, or back of the hand) and introducing a variety of different allergens. The other test involves injecting a small amount of allergen-containing solution just under the skin. If a weal (a raised area) and redness develop, you are allergic to the substance in question. After several hours or days, the irritation normally goes away. Although skin tests show that you are allergic to a particular substance, they do not necessarily indicate that the allergen causes asthma symptoms. The allergen may simply cause another allergic reaction, such as itching or teary eyes.

Which one of these tests is better? While the scratch test is not as sensitive, it tends to produce less intense reactions than the test involving injection. This is important if an exaggerated allergic response (known as *anaphylaxis*) is suspected. Anaphylactic reactions are never pleasant, but serious responses can sometimes involve fainting, shock, convulsions, and even death.

FOOD TESTS

You read earlier that certain foods can trigger asthma attacks in some individuals. Sometimes you know which foods these are, and they can be removed from the diet. However, since you normally choose from a wide variety of foods every day (and a recipe for a single dish can contain more than a dozen different ingredients), it is sometimes difficult to track down the food or foods that are asthma triggers.

The Food Challenge

You can often discover an asthma trigger in food by doing what is known as a *food challenge*. The food that is the suspected allergen is mixed with "safe" foods to disguise its presence. This will eliminate any psychological associations you may have about the food in question. If the food has a strong taste, an extract is placed in a capsule and swallowed during the meal. The doctor will then monitor your progress for several hours to see if a reaction takes place. This reaction can be an asthma flare, or reduced peak flow capacity as measured by a peak flow meter. Sometimes several days of monitoring will be necessary to determine food allergy through this method.

The Elimination Diet

This procedure involves excluding the food that is suspected of triggering asthma from your diet. If you are allergic to an obvious food such as shrimp or almonds, the test will be relatively easy. But if the suspected allergen is milk, you will have to eliminate all foods of milk origin (including yogurt, ice cream, and cheese) as well as any foods containing milk, such as bread, pastry, creamed soups, and puddings. You usually follow this type of elimination diet for several weeks. A more radical elimination diet involves eating only a few selected bland foods that do not trigger asthma, while excluding everything else. Over the next few weeks you gradually reintroduce the foods you normally consume, taking note of what foods are eaten and when. Peak flow measurements are taken several times daily while this diet is being followed. This type of diet can be a real hardship if you love to eat, but it will help you prevent asthma attacks in the long run. Remember that it should also be undertaken *only* under the supervision of a physician or registered dietitian.

DIAGNOSING THE ACUTE ATTACK

A final note on diagnosis. In the preceding pages we've spoken about the importance of an accurate and complete diagnosis by a physician. However, an acute asthma attack, while relatively uncommon, may not give you the luxury of taking the time to select a doctor and to go through the procedures we've already described. An acute attack can be life-threatening, and the sooner you recognize it, the faster you can seek proper medical care. While you shouldn't play doctor, you need to be aware that the presence of at least four of the following symptoms indicates that an acute asthma attack is taking place. Unless managed by asthma medication, they indicate that the patient requires immediate hospitalization:

1. A heart rate of 120 beats per minute (or twice the normal rate)

2. A respiratory rate of thirty or more breaths per minute (or twice the normal rate)

3. A peak expiratory flow rate of 120 liters per minute or less in adults (as determined by a peak flow reading)

4. Moderate or severe labored breathing

5. Moderate or severe wheezing

6. Need for the use of accessory muscles (such as those in the shoulders or neck) in addition to the chest muscles in order to breathe

Since many of these symptoms are best evaluated by a physician, an at-home diagnosis may not be the most accurate. However, it's better to err on the side of safety and go to your physician (or hospital emergency room) if you believe that you are experiencing an acute attack rather than let it continue uncontrolled.

THE NEXT STEP

After your physician discovers the trigger factors and determines the frequency and intensity of asthma, he or she creates an individualized treatment program for you. The treatment program has two major goals: to help prevent the onset of asthma attacks, and to manage an attack once it has begun.

In the following chapters we examine some successful home-care strategies to help prevent and manage asthma flares.

DRUG TREATMENT

Medical science has not been able to cure asthma. However, over the past twenty years there have been many important medical advances that can do much to control and treat your asthma symptoms. Through preventive care and aggressive symptom management, the vast majority of asthma patients today can live active, fulfilling lives.

There are two basic ways to treat asthma through medication: The symptoms themselves are relieved with drugs, or regular drug therapy is taken to help prevent symptoms from coming about. The physician's goal is to use the least amount of medication necessary to achieve the desired results.

DRUGS THAT RELIEVE SYMPTOMS: BRONCHODILATORS

Bronchodilators open up (dilate) narrowed airways (bronchioles). Some are available in tablet or syrup form, while most are taken through a special inhaler that brings the medicine directly into the bronchial tubes. This often involves the need for less medication than other delivery methods. As a result, there is a corresponding reduction in adverse side effects.

Generally speaking, these drugs are usually taken when you feel an attack coming on as well as during the attack itself. They come in the following three varieties.

Adrenergics

This class of bronchodilators works like adrenaline, a hormone produced by the adrenal gland. That is why they are known as adrenaline derivatives. They are also known in the medical profession as *beta-2 agonists*. These drugs have the ability to relax air passages and slow the release of histamine from the mast cells, and are considered the first drugs of choice by most physicians in this country to treat asthma symptoms. Adrenergic bronchodilators can be used in anticipation of an asthma flare (among patients with exercise-induced asthma, they are often used several minutes before physical activity) or during it. They have been found useful in mild, moderate, and severe asthma flares.

The generic and (in parentheses) the brand names of the most popular adrenergic bronchodilators include:

- albuterol (Proventil, Ventolin)

- metaproterenol (Alupent, Metaprel)

- terbutane (Bricanil, Brethine)

Adrenalin (epinephrine) is a synthetic hormone that enjoyed wide use before more advanced medications came along. However, it caused a wide variety of adverse side effects, especially for patients with hypertension, diabetes, glaucoma, or heart disease. At present it is not as widely prescribed by doctors, but is still available in some over-the-counter medications.

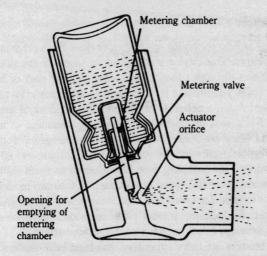

Figure 6-1. A metered dose inhaler.

Inhalers

The primary way to take adrenergic bronchodilators is through an *inhaler* or puffer. The metered dose inhaler, as seen in Figure 6-1, is the most popular. Like an aerosol container, its contents are under pressure, and the medicine is suspended in liquid. When a dose is needed, you press on the canister, and a measured dose of medication is released through the mouthpiece in the form of a fine spray. You then breathe the medicine directly into your lungs. Inhalers are inexpensive and portable. However, if you need an inhaler, get some instruction before using it. If you don't use it correctly, you won't get enough medicine into the lungs to be effective. Some younger and even older patients find the metered dose inhaler difficult to use. For these people, a variety of other inhalers is available.

Nebulizer

If your asthma is chronic or serious, doctors often recommend a nebulizer. This device involves an air pump or compressor that blows through a mouthpiece a fine aerosol mist of medicine, which you breathe in. Because it is more powerful than a regular inhaler, a nebulizer can deliver a larger dose of medication. Nebulizers are used for emergency treatment of acute asthma (they are found in most hospital emergency rooms), for regular treatment of patients with chronic or severe asthma, and for providing protective therapy to small children. There are two basic types of nebulizer. A tabletop model has been available for years and runs on ordinary house electric current. In addition, several portable models have recently been developed that run on a rechargeable battery.

Nebulizers are more expensive than hand-held inhalers, and since nebulizers deliver a higher dose of medication, their use can bring about more side effects. Consult with your physician before purchasing and using one of these machines.

Some bronchodilators can be taken in tablet or syrup form, and several (such as epinephrine) are injected.

Adverse Side Effects/Adverse Reactions Adrenergic bronchodilators may cause nausea, rapid heartbeat, throat discomfort, and tremor. In addition, beta-2 agonists can interact with certain other medications such as beta blockers, so patients taking other drugs should consult their physician regarding possible adverse interactions.

Anticholinergics

This second type of bronchodilator blocks the action of the vagus nerve and helps the bronchial muscles to relax when they are constricted. It also dries up mucus. The major medication of this type is known as ipratropium or Atrovent. It is primarily taken through an inhaler. This new drug is considered to have fewer side effects than atropine, an older anticholinergic bronchodilator used primarily to treat severe asthma cases.

Side Effects/Adverse Reactions Anticholinergic bronchodilators can bring about dry mouth, rapid heartbeat, dizziness, constipation, and urinary retention. There is also the potential for developing tolerance or increased airway reactivity if the use of Atrovent is abruptly discontinued.

Methylxanthines

This group of asthma medications is derived from caffeine. Like other bronchodilators, they are very effective in opening up the air passages during an asthma attack, and are also used when the patient feels that an asthma flare is coming on. They can be taken as a daily preventive medication.

The most common bronchodilator of this type is theophylline, which is sold under more than fifty different brand names. It is considered one of the most useful asthma drugs by American doctors, but it is not as widely used in Western Europe. In Europe (and especially in the United Kingdom) doctors place more emphasis on the use of inhaled steroids to prevent asthma flares. Theophylline is popular because a single dose of its new slow-release form can be effective for up to twelve hours, so it is useful in helping prevent cases of night asthma. However, it is not considered very effective during an asthma attack itself. Because theophylline brings about coughing if inhaled, it is mostly taken in tablet or liquid form.

It is important to monitor proper dosage of theophylline with the physician, because a number of factors—including a high-carbohydrate, low-protein diet; smoking; coffee; and certain other medications—can affect the level of theophylline in the blood. If the theophylline level in the blood is too low, its effectiveness is impaired. If the level is too high, the adverse reactions mentioned below can result.

Theophylline: Side Effects/Adverse Reactions   Major side effects of theophylline include restlessness, nervousness, upset stomach, headache, nausea, vomiting, loss of appetite, irregular heartbeat, heart palpitations, and convulsions.

If you take theophylline, you have to be careful to avoid taking any *myacin* drugs to control infections. Always ask your physician about possible adverse drug interactions if you require an antibiotic while you are taking asthma medications such as theophylline.

Combinations

Very often a combination of bronchodilators (one from each of two or three groups) is prescribed as one medicine. However, whether used alone or in combination, it is important to achieve the lowest dose of bronchodilator necessary to control symptoms. This is especially the case with children, because they are often more responsive to medications than adults. It has been well documented that less medication is needed *before* an attack than *during* one. This is why it is important to anticipate a potential problem before it actually takes place.

Achieving this is not always easy, and it requires careful monitoring by both you and your physician. For this reason, some doctors suggest that you keep a daily record on your health status. First, make a careful notation of peak flow readings several times a day, along with any symptoms and exposures to triggers (such as cat dander or cold air) that may have precipitated a flare during the day or night. Your record also includes any specific medications (and the dose) that were used to prevent or control the asthma flare. This enables the doctor to prescribe better the lowest dose necessary to manage asthma flares.

DRUGS THAT PREVENT SYMPTOMS

Corticosteroids

Steroids are used when you have frequent symptoms or experience wide variations in breathing (as measured by the peak-flow meter). For the most part, these medications are taken regularly whether you have asthma symptoms or not. The most widely used drugs are inhaled steroids, steroid tablets, and chromolyn sodium. At the time of this writing, there are more than twenty-five specific preventive asthma drugs and routes of delivery.

The term *steroid* includes a wide variety of hormones produced by the body. However, in our discussion of asthma we are dealing with a group of steroids known as *corticosteroids*. They are related to cortisone, the hormone produced by the adrenal gland to regulate the body's metabolism of protein, fat, carbohydrates, sodium, and potassium. Corticosteroids should not be confused with anabolic steroids, which are occasionally abused by athletes to increase their muscle mass.

Corticosteroids are valuable in asthma treatment because in addition to preventing asthma symptoms from appearing, they relieve wheezing like bronchodilators do. Corticosteroids reduce the swelling of the air passages resulting from inflammation, and they reduce mucus as well. They also can enhance the effect of certain bronchodilators. Steroids are used primarily by patients with chronic or severe asthma, especially when bronchodilator therapy has not been effective. For many asthma sufferers, steroids have enabled them to live normal lives. However, because steroids can have many adverse side effects, the primary goal is to use only the minimal amount needed to control symptoms and to taper off use of the medication as soon as possible.

Steroids are either taken in tablet form or are inhaled. Oral steroids are powerful drugs and are prescribed for individuals with serious, chronic asthma, while in North America inhaled steroids have traditionally been recommended for less serious cases. However, in Europe they have long been used by a wide variety of asthma patients.

Oral Steroids

The most commonly used oral steroids in tablet form include prednisone (Meticorten), prednisolone (Deltacortef), methyl prednisolone (Medrol), and dexamethasone (Decadron). In haled steroids include beclomethasone (Vanceril, Beclovent) triamicinolone (Azmacort), and flunisolide (Aerobid).

Corticosteroids are prescribed for both long- and short-term use. A short-term "burst" of steroids (usually lasting three to five days) is used when asthma becomes very severe. When used for a short time, side effects are minimal, and use of the drug does not have to be tapered off when discontinuing its use is indicated. For patients who are unable to control their asthma with bronchodilators alone, long-term steroid use is often recommended. They are taken either orally or through an inhaler and are used primarily every day or every other day

Side Effects/Adverse Reactions When taken over the short term, oral steroids can produce mood swings, weight gain, swelling due to edema (water retention), and elevated blood pressure. Their long-term use is associated with more serious side effects. These include slow wound healing and poor resistance to infection, osteoporosis, peptic ulcer, and loss of potassium and calcium. Other side effects can include high blood pressure, cataracts, weight gain, mood swings, and depression. Susceptible individuals can develop diabetes and heart disease. Long-term oral steroid use can also inhibit the growth rate of children. If their use is abruptly discontinued, oral steroids can trigger an asthma attack.

Inhaled Steroids

Although not as potent, inhaled steroids are considered safer than oral steroids. Because the inhaler delivers medication directly to where it is needed, less medication is required. Inhaled steroids also have relatively few adverse side effects, and their use can be discontinued without tapering off.

Side Effects/Adverse Reactions   Adverse reactions from the use of inhaled steroids include sore throat due to thrush, and huskiness or hoarseness of the voice. You can alleviate these problems by rinsing your mouth with water or gargling with mouthwash after each use.

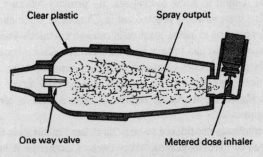

Figure 6-2. Inhaler with spacer device.

Some doctors recommend use of a *spacer* or holding chamber (see Figure 6-2), which catches the dose from a metered-dose inhaler and holds it until the patient starts to breathe in. Rather than forcing the mist into the respiratory tract, it allows the medication to be breathed in at a slower rate. Because they are effective and cause minimal side effects, inhaled steroids are often the drug of choice among European physicians to prevent asthma flares. They have not been used widely in North America.

It is important to remember that everyone who takes steroids to control asthma will not necessarily experience every one of the adverse reactions mentioned above. However, if any occur, it is a good idea to speak to your physician about them. He or she may be able to offer suggestions on how the side effects can be minimized. Consult the excellent book *Asthma* by Allan M. Weinstein, M.D., for a more detailed discussion about using steroids and other asthma medications.

Cromolyn

Cromolyn (Intal) is a relatively new preventive medication that can be helpful to some individuals. Its primary function is to stabilize mast cells. As pointed out in Chapter 2, when affected by allergens or irritants, mast cells release chemicals (such as histamines) that can trigger an asthma attack. Cromolyn inhibits this process, even after the person is exposed to an allergen (such as pollen) or an irritant (such as cold air or exercise). However, it cannot reduce an attack that is already taking place.

Cromolyn is considered to be a "first line" medication for all degrees of chronic asthma. Many doctors prescribe it before recommending long-term steroid use. It is inhaled into the lungs through a variety of inhaler devices, and both the dose and technique of delivery into the lungs should be precise.

Side Effects/Adverse Reactions   Cromolyn has very few side effects, especially when compared to other asthma medications. Adverse reactions can include cough, throat irritation, and tightening of the air passages. It is also not recommended for pregnant women.

Combination Therapies

In recent years, asthma doctors have been placing more emphasis on combination therapies. These involve the use of, for example, a bronchodilator along with a preventive medication such as cromolyn or an inhaled steroid. Another combination used primarily for patients with severe asthma and who are taking steroids involves use of an antibiotic (antibiotics are normally used to treat infectious diseases) known as troleandomycin (TAO) combined with methylprednisolone (Medrol), an oral steroid. By combining these two drugs it has been found that an overall lower dose of steroid is required.

When prescribing a combination of medications to control asthma, your doctor needs to be aware of any additional drugs you may be taking in order to avoid potentially harmful drug interactions.

Allergy Shots

Allergy shots are composed of small doses of a substance (an allergen) that you are allergic to. You are injected with the allergen so that your body will be less sensitive to it in the future. Allergy shots are mostly given to individuals who have a proven allergen that triggers asthma, as well as to people with multiple allergies that result in year-round symptoms. They are also used by people who are unable to control their allergic asthma through other medications. Allergy shots are not for everyone, but have been found to help many who suffer primarily from allergic reactions due to pollen and dust. An average allergy shot program lasts three to five years.

Because strong adverse reactions are possible when an allergen such as animal dander is injected, many allergists suggest removing the animal rather than taking the shot.

Side Effects/Adverse Reactions   The most common adverse reaction to allergy shots is redness and inflammation of the region surrounding the injection site. This usually disappears after a few days. However, in some individuals an *anaphylactic* or exaggerated allergic reaction is possible. This can involve shock, fever, and convulsions. Severe attacks may even result in death.

OVER-THE-COUNTER ASTHMA MEDICATIONS

Within the past few years a number of asthma medications have become publicly available without a prescription. Some have been heavily advertised on television and in magazines. The most popular are products containing epinephrine, a bronchodilator that has been used to treat asthma symptoms for many years.

Some physicians feel that when over-the-counter products containing epinephrine are used properly, they can be helpful in managing occasional, short-term, mild asthma symptoms. Because it is a nonprescription drug, epinephrine is administered in a smaller dose than is usually found in prescribed epinephrine. As a result, it relieves symptoms for a relatively short time. Unfortunately, this can lead to a tendency for the asthma patient to use it over and over to control asthma flares. Doctors warn that frequent, repeated use can not only cause dependency on the drug but also may cause you to put off getting needed medical attention. If the person with asthma is already taking other medications—whether for asthma or another health problem—the addition of epinephrine can produce harmful interactions with certain other drugs. According to Dr. Malcolm Hill of the National Jewish Center for Immunology and Respiratory Medicine, it is better to address the basic issues of the disease (including having a thorough diagnosis, discovering trigger factors, and developing aggressive doctor-patient asthma management) than merely treating the symptoms. If you are an asthma patient (or feel that you might be suffering from asthma symptoms), common sense dictates that you consult your physician before taking a nonprescription asthma drug.

Other asthma medications are being developed. Some of the major ones are described in Chapter 12, "The Future of Asthma Management."

EFFECTIVE PATIENT MANAGEMENT

When taking a bronchodilator, steroid, or any other prescribed asthma medication, you have to take it at the right times and in the correct amounts. Doctors report that most of the asthma cases that have been difficult to manage have a single component: The patient did not monitor his or her condition and did not take the medications that were prescribed in the correct doses. This may be due to a wide variety of factors, including lack of family support, inability to administer the drugs effectively, or unpleasant side effects caused by the drugs. For example, some medications cause depression and mood swings. As a result, patients are less likely to make the effort to take these medications.

Ultimately it is your responsibility to work—in partnership with your physician—to achieve an effective program of asthma care and management. In addition to learning everything possible about asthma, its causes, and its treatment, you and your physician must develop a regimen that fits into your life-style, one that must include the following components to be effective:

1. Instructions on effective self-monitoring

2. Written explanations of what you have been taught at the doctor's office or hospital

3. Specific times at which medications should be taken

4. *Complete* and *clear* explanations of possible side effects

Studies at major health centers and hospitals have shown that patients who take a passive role and don't feel that they are in control of their care tend to feel frustrated and helpless in dealing with their condition. As a result, they are not able to manage their asthma successfully. The same studies show that patients who take a more active role in their care are not only better able to prevent and control their symptoms but tend to feel better about themselves as well.

If you are taking medications for more than one health problem, be especially aware of possible negative interactions with asthma drugs. For example, certain epilepsy drugs interact negatively with some asthma medications, as can drugs taken for diabetes, heart disease, or other lung problems. If you have asthma but are seeing a different physician for another health problem, tell each doctor about the other medications you are taking. As an extra precaution, it's a good idea to obtain your medications from *the same pharmacy* so that your pharmacist can determine if any of the drugs you are taking may interreact in a negative way.

A final note: While today's asthma medications can be very useful in the prevention and treatment of asthma symptoms, using them more often than prescribed (or in progressively larger doses) often indicates that the asthma is not under control. Other danger signs include more frequent and more severe episodes of wheezing or shortness of breath, increased shortness of breath while walking or climbing stairs, a reduction in your peak expiratory flow rate as measured by the peak-flow meter, and an increasing difference between your morning and evening peak-flow readings. If any of these problems is noted, consult your physician. If subsequently there is still no improvement, you may need to see another doctor.

SEVEN

CONTROLLING YOUR ENVIRONMENT

What can you do to make your life easier as an asthma patient? We've seen that medication is effective in helping to minimize and manage your symptoms but clearly it is far better to prevent symptoms from occurring in the first place. Although the list of environmental trigger factors is long, the good news is that most people with asthma react only to several of them. Let's see how we can reduce exposure to allergens and irritants in and around the home, at work, and while traveling. (We will deal with food-related allergens and irritants in the following chapter, on diet.)

For the vast majority of asthma patients, asthma triggers can be identified and controlled. This involves becoming a keen observer of your environment and being aware of the types of triggers that affect you during the day or night. Some triggers—such as cigarette smoke—may be fairly obvious. Others may require taking a series of blood or skin tests for possible allergy. In his excellent book *Asthma,* Dr. Allan M. Weinstein suggests that a daily record of one's movements and asthma symptoms during the day is useful, because it can reveal any delayed reactions to trigger factors in the environment. Although these methods require time and effort, they are valuable in the long run because by discovering what the trigger factors are, we can learn how to limit our exposure to them.

POLLEN

For most people with asthma, *pollen* is a major trigger of allergy and asthma symptoms. As we mentioned in Chapter 2, pollen, a fine powder produced by flowers, fertilizes other flowers of the same species. The amount of pollen in the air varies in different parts of the country and also varies according to the season. For example, during May there is a higher pollen count in the Pocono Mountains of Pennsylvania than in the semiarid Sandia Mountains of New Mexico.

During the day, pollen rises toward the sky, and it descends at night. To limit exposure to pollen while you are indoors, open windows during the middle of the day only. It is also good to have double-glazed windows, particularly in the bedroom. For many asthma patients, the bedroom should be designated their safe room—one that is as free from allergens as possible. Air conditioning (especially with the filters of the unit replaced regularly) is also a recommended way to reduce pollen within the home.

Of course, we cannot remain indoors indefinitely. If you are sensitive to pollen, try to go outdoors during those times of the day when the pollen count is down, and try to move about in an air-conditioned vehicle. Before leaving the house you can also take medications that can help prevent an asthma flare. When you return home it is a good idea to rinse your hair, especially before going to bed at night. This may help avoid asthma attacks at night due to pollen that you may bring into the house. Pets should be kept outside during the pollen season so that they don't bring pollen indoors.

When pollen is a trigger of asthma symptoms, vacations can become a real ordeal. Since pollen poses few problems during the winter, ski vacations and trips to snowy areas can be very enjoyable for asthma patients who are allergic to pollen. However, during the warmer months, vacations in high elevations or in places receiving offshore breezes are often recommended for people who are allergic to pollen, simply because there is less of it in the air there.

MOLDS

The microscopic spores released into the air by *molds* (or mildew) make up another common asthma trigger. As we pointed out earlier, molds naturally occur in warm and humid places, both inside and outside the home.

The bathroom. Clean your shower curtains, porcelain fixtures, closets, and hard-to-get areas regularly and thoroughly. Use a fungicide if necessary. However, avoid any aerosol cleaners as well as bathroom cleansers containing ammonia, pine oil, or petrochemicals.

The bedroom. Air out your sheets and blankets regularly, except during the pollen season (unless you know that you are absolutely not allergic to pollen). Because we often perspire at night, pillows can become damp over time. For this reason they should be replaced every few years. In all rooms, avoid using heavy carpets; replace them with light rugs, or simply keep the bare floors polished and clean. Remove all damp wall paper, and paint the walls. It is also important to replace foam upholstery regularly to avoid mildew. Clean kitchen wastebaskets regularly.

Dehumidifiers? Some allergists suggest that a dehumidifier is useful when humidity rises above a certain level, especially in the basement. However, dehumidifiers can be areas of mold growth themselves, so filters need to be changed regularly. Fans are also suggested to keep air moving indoors. However, when using a fan, the house must be relatively dust-free.

Outdoors. Major sources of mold spores outdoors include compost heaps, blocked rainwater channels, freshly cut grass, and even a pile of sand against an outside wall. Of course, eliminating mold-producing sources like a blocked rainwater gutter is important. In place of grass, some people have found that a Japanese garden, made primarily of gravel and stone, is an effective (and attractive) way to reduce asthma symptoms caused by grass. In place of grass, a variety of shrubs can be planted to provide beauty outside the home. They often require a minimum of care.

DUST

Of all allergens, *dust* is one of the most troublesome for asthma patients. As we mentioned earlier, dust comes not only from outside the home, but also from dead skin, food fragments, animal dander or dandruff, and microscopic particles of cloth. For sensitive people with asthma, it is not the dust itself that causes allergy but the microscopic feces of the house dust mite, which thrives on the dust in the home.

Get rid of dust. For most people, the best way to avoid dust accumulation in the home is to clean it regularly. The bedroom should be cleaned twice a week (especially the closet), and floors in other rooms should be cleaned at least once a week. Although a vacuum cleaner is effective in removing dust, it tends to blow dust around as well. For this reason, dusting with a damp cloth is preferable. It's also a good idea to avoid items that are likely to collect dust, such as ornate items, heavy drapes, knickknacks, stuffed animals, and heavy carpets. Since books often are dust collectors, use an enclosed bookshelf rather than one where the books are exposed. Generally speaking, use closed storage facilities whenever possible rather than open shelves.

Use artificial fibers. Dust mites love natural fibers. To help achieve a mite-free environment, use artificial fibers in bedding, carpets, curtains, and stuffed animals. Latex foam mattresses and Dacron pillows are especially recommended. Some asthma patients avoid traditional mattresses completely and choose a water bed instead. It is also a good idea to enclose mattresses, box springs, and pillows in an allergenproof casing. Nonslip casings are now becoming more readily available in many retail outlets.

Air cleaners. Air cleaners can help keep a home dust-free. The most recommended filter is the high-efficiency particulate air (HEPA) filter, because it can eliminate nearly 100 percent of all airborne particles in the home. Dehumidifiers are also useful, since mites cannot live when the humidity is under 50 percent. However, if humidity drops too low, your nasal passages may dry out and breathing may become uncomfortable.

Should you move? A more radical solution to the dust mite problem is to move to an elevation of thirty-six hundred feet or higher. Mites (as well as most types of mold) cannot survive at that altitude.

ANIMALS

Pets can be a problem for some people with asthma. Humans have been found to be allergic to a wide variety of animals, including cats, dogs, horses, guinea pigs, birds, and hamsters. Although children often become emotionally involved with pets, they also tend to develop allergies to domestic animals more than adults do.

Male animals tend to cause more allergies than female animals, and different breeds can have a more pronounced allergic effect. For example, Persian and Siamese cats tend to trigger asthma more than other breeds, and short-haired dogs cause more allergic reactions than long-haired dogs do.

In dogs and horses, dander or dandruff seems to be the primary asthma trigger, while among cats, both dander and saliva are the main culprits. The feathers of birds (whether on the bird or in pillows) are also allergenic. Urine is a common allergen of rodents such as hamsters, white mice, and guinea pigs. While few people keep cockroaches as pets, they tend to become uninvited residents in homes and apartments, especially in larger cities. In the case of roaches, the primary allergen is their feces.

Although it's often a heartbreaking decision, the most effective solution to avoid asthma trigger factors caused by pets is to remove the animal from the home. This is recommended especially when asthma due to animals is severe. In milder cases the pet must be kept out of the bedroom, which, as mentioned before, should always be a haven for the asthma sufferer. Although they tend not to be as responsive as a cat or a dog, fish or reptiles make good pets and do not trigger asthma symptoms.

ALLERGIES AND IRRITANTS IN THE WORKPLACE

It is believed that over two hundred substances in the workplace can trigger asthma symptoms. In some professions such as farming or carpentry, the particular trigger can be easily identified. In other professions (such as those involved in the petrochemical industry) it may be more difficult.

Though not always easy to carry out, here are some basic strategies for dealing with identified occupational allergens:

1. Substitute a less toxic product for the substance that is triggering your asthma.

2. Eradicate or avoid the substance through standard procedures of industrial cleanliness. To do this, you may need to enlist the help of your supervisor or union.

3. Use a face mask on the job if you cannot avoid working with the offending substance.

4. Take a bronchodilator or other medication to prevent an attack from taking place.

5. Switch to another job function at work that doesn't require contact with the allergenic substance. A doctor's note may be needed to help you do this.

6. If all else fails, you may have to leave your job altogether, and seek employment in a field where you are not exposed to allergens that can trigger your asthma.

AIR POLLUTION

As we mentioned in Chapter 2, air pollutants can be powerful triggers for asthma attack. The three major types of environmental pollution include sulfur dioxide; ozone; and nitrogen dioxide, a major component of cigarette smoke.

In a world of increasing pollution, it is difficult to avoid it completely. We have to try to live as normal a life as possible, and fortunately most asthma patients—especially those with mild to moderate asthma that is under control—can lead a normal life unless pollution is severe.

However, when the pollution has reached unhealthy levels, you can protect yourself through the following simple strategies:

1. Stay indoors. By keeping windows closed and turning on the air conditioner, your chances of avoiding pollutants are better than walking around outside or letting polluted air enter the house.

2. Avoid using gas ranges, since burning gas creates nitrogen dioxide. If you must cook with gas, use a kitchen exhaust fan.

3. If you have to go outside during an inversion or a time of severe pollution, allergists recommend pretreatment with a bronchodilator. While not a foolproof method of prevention, it may help diminish the chances of an asthma flare.

4. If you suffer from asthma, avoid cigarette smoke as much as possible at *all* times.

For some sensitive individuals, certain perfumes and other odors can trigger asthma. This is why it is important to avoid all strong perfumes, especially when walking past perfume counters in department stores. Household cleansers with strong odors can be replaced by those without added perfume. Kitchen odors can be eliminated to a large extent by using an exhaust fan while cooking.

ON THE ROAD

If you travel by car, here are some tips to help you enjoy your journey.

1. For many people with asthma, the automobile—provided that windows are closed—can be a good refuge from pollen, dust, and air pollution.

2. Air conditioning is also useful in reducing exposure to pollen and other airborne irritants, especially if the filters are changed regularly.

3. It is a good idea always to carry a peak-flow meter, asthma medication, and metered dose inhaler when you travel by automobile. Portable nebulizers can also be carried in the car and plugged into the cigarette lighter if required.

IN THE AIR

Air travel is considered relatively safe for people with mild asthma. Nevertheless, here are a few suggestions:

1. On international flights, choose a seat in the section for nonsmokers; the seat should be as far from the smoking area as possible. In the United States, smoking is now prohibited on all domestic flights.

2. Since a reduction of oxygen normally occurs during jet travel, asthma patients whose symptoms include a reduction of oxygen in the blood should consult with their physician before traveling by air.

3. As with automobile travel, take your peak-flow meter, inhaler, and medication with you on the plane. If you suffer from severe asthma, carry a portable nebulizer on board as well. Before the plane leaves the gate, inform the flight attendant that you suffer from asthma, in case you need assistance during the flight.

MOVING

Some asthma patients take the radical step of moving to another part of the country to avoid allergens. Phoenix, Arizona, and Denver, Colorado, used to be the most popular destinations for people with asthma who couldn't put up with the pollen of the East or the Midwest. Many people moved without even being sure that their asthma was triggered by pollen or other environmental factors common in the East, and were disappointed when their asthma failed to lessen.

The high air pollution of cities such as Denver and Phoenix has largely eliminated this option. In addition, many new residents in places such as Arizona have brought plants common in the East with them to create a more familiar atmosphere. Instead of sand and cacti, their homes are surrounded by lawns and flowering plants that are native to the East or Midwest. As a result, the pollens from these plants affect people with asthma as if they had never left their homes in New Jersey or Indiana.

Although it is sometimes possible to find a new region of the country that is relatively free of the offending substance, allergists point out that new allergies can develop at any time. Some may be worse than the original. They suggest that it is better to do everything possible to control asthma through preventive medication and environmental control first. If these measures fail, your physician may be able to suggest areas in the country that may be better suited to your needs. However, before you actually move to another region to avoid asthma triggers, spend a few weeks visiting the area and monitor any adverse reactions to the environment.

Moving to another part of the country (or the world) is a radical decision, and should be discussed at length with both your physician and with all family members who would be affected by such a move.

EIGHT

DIET

If you suffer from asthma, eating well may be a problem for you. Some asthma patients are allergic to certain foods, while others (especially those taking steroids) may not be getting enough of the nutrients they need.

FOOD ALLERGY AND ASTHMA

Many asthma patients automatically assume that they must adopt very restricted diets to avoid asthma flares. They imagine they must avoid wheat, corn, nuts, smoked meats, milk, eggs, cheese, beer, wine, canned juices, and a host of other "no's." Needless to say, this belief often leads to an overall feeling of deprivation and desperation, and makes the lot of the asthma patient a most unhappy one.

If you have asthma that you suspect may be diet-related, take a more positive approach. In the first place, you need to find out which foods may be bad for you and which are not. Instead of banning all suspected foods, take the time to identify systematically the food or foods to which you are actually allergic. Rather than avoid a much-loved food because it is *suspected* of triggering asthma, find out for sure. Nutritionists suggest that a physician-supervised food challenge test (as described in Chapter 5) is the best way to find out what the offending food really is. Although food challenge tests and elimination diets may be inconvenient and time-consuming in the short run, they will make your life far easier over the long term.

Multiple Food Allergies

Recent findings indicate that among people whose asthma is triggered by diet, far fewer have multiple food allergies than was previously believed. It is also interesting to note that a study of children with food allergies found that approximately 60 percent of those who suffer from food-related allergies are allergic to only one or two allergens in food, 30 percent are allergic to three, and only 10 percent of the children in the study are allergic to four or more.

WHAT TO WATCH OUT FOR

If you suspect that asthma is triggered by diet, the foods most likely to be responsible for food allergy include:

• cow's milk (among young children)

• eggs

• wheat and other cereals

• certain seafoods

• certain types of nuts

Remember that you may be allergic to only *one* kind of nut or *one* kind of cereal. For example, a breakfast cereal containing wheat may be bad for you, while one containing corn may be okay. This is why an elimination diet or a food challenge test (described in Chapter 5) can help.

In addition, there are a number of elements added to foods that you may need to be concerned about.

SULFITES

A small minority of asthma patients are allergic to chemical additives known as sulfites. As we mentioned earlier, sulfiting agents (including sodium and potassium bisulfite, sodium and potassium metabisulfite, sulfur dioxide, and sodium sulfite) are routinely added to foods to prevent the appearance of spoilage when they are exposed to air. Sulfiting agents retard browning and generally help foods maintain a fresh, just-picked appearance.

Sulfites are sometimes added to fresh fruits and vegetables in markets, especially when they are cut up and placed on display. They are also added to shrimp and seafood. Bakeries sometimes use sulfites as dough conditioners, and some food manufacturers add them to bread and cake mixes. Delicatessens and restaurants often add sulfites to foods offered in salad bars to maintain a fresh appearance when the foods are on display all day. Some restaurants add sulfites to peeled or raw potatoes that are waiting to be cooked to keep them looking white. Caterers routinely add sulfites to fresh fruits and vegetables as well.

Many manufactured foods contain sulfites. In the food processing industry, sulfites help retard spoilage due to microbes, minimize browning and discoloration, inhibit the formation of undesirable microorganisms in fermentation, and are used to sanitize equipment used in the fermentation of foods.

Specific Foods Containing Sulfites

- dried fish

- shrimp and other types of shellfish

- fresh grapes (primarily those from California)

- dried fruits (especially those light in color, such as apricots, pears, and apples)

- commercially prepared bread

- bread and pastry that contains dried fruits

- dehydrated or instant potatoes

- products containing dehydrated vegetables (including soup mixes, salad dressings, and food mixes)

- seasonings containing dehydrated vegetables

- some brands of soft drinks, wine, and beer

Avoiding Sulfites

The best way to avoid sulfites in restaurants is to ask your waiter. Over the past few years, restaurant owners have become more aware of the needs of people allergic to sulfites and are eager to accommodate them. It is also important to read the labels of commercially manufactured food products to see if one or more of the sulfiting agents listed above are used. Although there can be no guarantees, breads, pastries, soup mixes, and dried fruits sold in natural-food stores are more likely to be sulfite-free than those found in ordinary supermarkets. Wherever you buy processed foods, read the labels.

FOOD COLORING AND OTHER ADDITIVES

In addition to sulfites, a number of other food additives can trigger an asthma flare in sensitive people. These substances must be listed on food labels, so be sure to examine the list of ingredients before you buy.

Yellow Food Dye No. 5 (Tartrazine)

Tartrazine is sometimes added to cookies, cakes, pudding mixes, syrups, and soft drinks. It is also used in some prescribed and over-the-counter medications. It is even found in some asthma medications. Check with your pharmacist.

Monosodium Glutamate

Monosodium glutamate (or MSG) can be a potent trigger of asthma attack. An additive that has been used for thousands of years, MSG is commonly used in Chinese restaurants as a flavor enhancer. It is also used as a preservative in many processed foods. Read grocery labels carefully.

Aspertame

As a sugar substitute marketed under the name Nutrasweet, aspertame is found in a wide variety of diet soft drinks, prepared desserts, and other diet foods.

A GOOD, BASIC DIET

Whether you have asthma or not, a good, well-balanced diet should be the foundation of your life. It should feature variety, moderation, and balance compatible with your taste, life-style, activity, and other individual needs. There is no one diet for everyone, and this section should not be considered a complete guide to achieving optimum nutrition. However, most experts believe that a healthful diet is generally low in fat, refined sugar, salt, and heavily processed foods. It will probably contain fewer animal products than you are accustomed to, yet it will provide sufficient vitamins, minerals, proteins, dietary fiber, and other food elements essential for good health. A healthful diet should, of course, also be free from known asthma triggers such as sulfiting agents and certain other food additives. These substances will vary depending on the individual, since there are no known asthma triggers that are universal.

Many nutritionists suggest that we adopt the following recommendations offered in *Dietary Guidelines for Americans,* published by the U.S. Department of Agriculture and the U.S. Department of Health and Human Services in 1985:

• Eat a variety of foods.

• Maintain desirable weight.

• Avoid too much fat, saturated fat, and cholesterol.

• Eat foods with adequate starch and fiber.

• Avoid too much sugar.

• Avoid too much sodium.

• If you drink alcoholic beverages, do so in moderation.

These guidelines are considered very conservative and tend to leave much to interpretation. For clarity we will examine these recommendations in detail.

Eat a Variety of Foods

For a well-balanced diet, include fruits, vegetables, whole-grain cereals, enriched breads, and a source of dairy products (such as low-fat milk, cheese, or yogurt) daily. Fish, lean meats, poultry, and eggs are considered complete proteins because they contain the nine essential amino acids, known as the building blocks of protein. Dried beans, lentils, peas, nuts, and seeds are also good sources of protein but do not contain all of the amino acids by themselves. For this reason they are called incomplete proteins. However, by combining them with other foods (such as rice and legumes, peanut butter and bread, wheat and legumes, legumes and seeds, cornmeal and beans, or wheat and soy), a complete protein can easily be achieved.

Maintain Desirable Weight

By eating food slowly and chewing it carefully, taking smaller portions and avoiding second helpings, and eating fewer fatty foods and less sugar, sweets, and alcoholic beverages, we can maintain control over the number of calories we consume. In place of these foods, we should consume fresh fruits, vegetables, and whole grains. Finally, by increasing physical activity we burn up more calories.

Avoid Too Much Fat, Saturated Fat, and Cholesterol

Fried foods, fatty meats, butter, cream, lard, some types of margarine, palm oil, and coconut oil are all high in fat, and their consumption should be reduced. Some margarines are high in hydrogenated fats, which are highly saturated, so be sure to read labels. In general monounsaturated oils such as olive oil and rapeseed (Puritan) oil are considered healthiest. But remember, your intake of all fats—even healthful ones—should be reduced.

Eggs and organ meats (such as liver) are high in protein, vitamins, and minerals but are also very high in cholesterol. For this reason they should be eaten sparingly. Lean meat, fish, poultry, and legumes (such as dried beans, peas, peanuts, soy products, and lentils) tend to be lower in fat and are recommended protein sources. Steam, bake, or broil your food rather than fry it. However, too much charbroiling may interfere with theophylline levels.

Eat Foods with Adequate Starch and Fiber

Good sources of fiber and starch (complex carbohydrates) include whole-grain breads and cereals (including oat and wheat bran); whole-grain pasta; fresh fruits and vegetables; and dry legumes such as peas, beans, and lentils.

Avoid Too Much Sugar

In addition to reducing obvious sources of sugar such as table sugar (white or brown), molasses, and honey, be aware that hidden sources of sugar find their way into a myriad of consumer products, such as cookies; crackers; cakes; beverages (including fruit punch, juice, and soft drinks); canned fruits, vegetables, and soups; and breakfast cereals. If the ingredients listed on the label begin with sugar, fructose, dextrose, glucose, or corn syrup, much of the product is made up of sugar. Read the labels.

Avoid Too Much Sodium

Like sugar, sodium is consumed in excess by most North Americans in the form of table salt. Before you add salt to the food you are cooking or eating, remember that many products, including potato chips, frozen dinners, pickled foods, soy sauce, processed cheese spreads, salted nuts, and canned soups and vegetables contain salt added by the manufacturer. Read the labels. By keeping your consumption of processed foods low, you will be more able to control sodium intake. Finally, in addition to limiting the amount of salt you add to foods, learn to use herbs and spices as substitutes.

If You Drink Alcoholic Beverages, Do So in Moderation

Alcoholic beverages are generally high in calories and low in nutrients. People who consume large quantities of alcohol run the risk of addiction, overweight, and vitamin and mineral deficiencies. When consumed by pregnant women, alcohol also has been linked to birth defects. Nutritionists tend to agree that one or two drinks per day do no harm to average adults (providing they are not pregnant and are not allergic to sulfites). Twelve ounces of beer, three and a half ounces of wine, and an ounce and a half of whiskey, rum, or vodka count as one drink.

VITAMIN AND MINERAL SUPPLEMENTS?

Because so much of today's foods are transported large distances, stored, and refined, they often do not arrive at the table with the amount of nutrients they had originally. For this reason, nutritionists often recommend a good daily vitamin and mineral supplement containing a wide range of nutrients for vitamin and mineral insurance. However, some registered dietitians find that an excessive intake of certain vitamins and minerals can decrease the body's absorption of other nutrients. This is why many are opposed to megavitamin therapy but recommend instead that approximately 100 percent of the recommended dietary allowance for nutrients is all that is needed from a multivitamin supplement.

SPECIAL NEEDS

Some asthma patients have special needs because the long-term use of steroids can interfere with the normal absorption and utilization of a number of important nutrients, including calcium, potassium, protein, vitamin C, and vitamin D. Steroid use can also cause you to retain other nutrients in your body, such as sodium.

Calcium

Calcium is a primary ingredient in bones. In addition to nutritional supplements (a suggested daily intake is one thousand to fifteen hundred milligrams), calcium intake can easily be increased by adding more milk products to the diet. (A cup of milk, for example, contains approximately three hundred milligrams of calcium, while a three-ounce serving of cheddar cheese provides 750 milligrams.) Calcium is also found in green vegetables such as kale, collards, and mustard greens, although the oxalic acid present in these foods inhibits calcium absorption. Calcium is also found in almonds and sunflower seeds.

Potassium

Potassium is a mineral that regulates muscle contraction and plays a role in the conduction of nerve impulses. Nutritionists suggest that in addition to maintaining a well-balanced diet, people who take steroids should consume two good sources of potassium daily. These include oranges and orange juice, apricots, cantaloupe, bananas, tomatoes, and baked potatoes.

Protein

Protein helps maintain strong muscles and also helps the body resist infection. In addition to meat and cheese, good protein sources include dried beans, lentils, soy products (including tofu, tempeh, and soybean meat analogs), nuts, and seeds. Since most North Americans consume far more protein than is recommended by the National Academy of Sciences, getting enough protein is not a problem for most asthma patients.

Vitamin C

This vitamin is essential for building strong bones and helps fight off infection. A well-balanced diet should contain several servings daily of citrus fruits and juices, melons, berries, or tomatoes. Broccoli, brussels sprouts, and green peppers are also good sources of vitamin C.

Vitamin D

Vitamin D promotes the normal calcification of bones and teeth. It is manufactured by the skin in the presence of sunlight. In addition to adequate exposure to sunshine, sources of this vitamin include fish liver oils, butter, and eggs. It is also added to milk. Rather than take a special supplement of vitamin D, nutritionists at the National Jewish Center for Immunology and Respiratory Medicine suggest that it be taken as part of a single multivitamin supplement for those patients who have problems consuming a normal balanced diet.

Sodium

Sodium is an essential component of most body fluids. However, it is often consumed in excess, and is linked with fluid retention and possibly high blood pressure. Use of steroids tends to make the body retain sodium. For this reason, nutritionists recommend that people taking steroids limit their intake of sodium to not more than three thousand milligrams per day. This would involve avoiding added salt, as well as many convenience foods, salted snack foods (such as potato chips, pretzels, and salted nuts), and many frozen food dinners.

Check the food labels for sodium content. Use sodium-free seasonings to flavor your food.

Just because you may have asthma that is triggered by certain foods, this doesn't mean that you can't enjoy eating. First, find out exactly what foods trigger your asthma; then find suitable substitutes that won't bring about allergic reactions. Experiment with cuisines from other countries, using foods that are safe. Check out some of the numerous cookbooks especially written for people with food allergies. They often contain recipes for delicious dishes that make eating for health eating for pleasure.

NINE

EXERCISE

Athletes with asthma have excelled in competitive sports. In fact, sixty-seven members of the U.S. Olympic Team at the 1984 summer Olympics in Los Angeles suffered from exercise-induced bronchospasm at one time or another. Thirty-eight of them won a total of forty-one medals, including fifteen gold, twenty-one silver, and five bronze! Some well-known Olympic athletes who have suffered from asthma include runner Jackie Joyner-Kersee, relay runner Jeanette Bolden, skier Bill Koch, long-distance runner Jim Ryun, and swimmer Nancy Hogshead.

In the past people with asthma were advised to avoid exercise and physical exertion as much as possible, but today a growing number of asthma specialists teach that the vast majority of asthma patients can safely participate in a wide variety of physical activities. This new viewpoint is due in part to a better awareness of the mechanics of exercise-related asthma itself, as well as to the development of drugs such as bronchodilators and cromolyn, which can prevent and manage asthma flares triggered by exercise and other strenuous physical activity.

Although an estimated eight of ten asthma patients feel some tightness in the chest during periods of vigorous physical activity, exercise-induced bronchospasm does not affect every asthma patient. Nearly everyone tends to get out of breath after a period of strenuous exercise, but if you experience wheezing or coughing during or after exercise, it may be a triggering factor for you. Your physician can confirm this suspicion by carrying out a breathing test before and after a period of exercise to measure your peak-flow rate. If the peak-flow rate is low after the exercise has stopped, your asthma is triggered by exercise.

This does not necessarily mean that you cannot exercise. It is now widely known that the benefits of exercise far outweigh any risks to most asthma patients, especially if the exercises are performed with care and involve good preventive strategies. Let's look at some of the benefits of exercise for asthma patients and examine the best (and the worst) exercises to choose from. We will also draw from the expertise of exercise and rehabilitation therapists at the National Jewish Center for Immunology and Respiratory Medicine in Denver, and discuss how people with asthma can achieve optimal fitness with minimum difficulty.

EXERCISE-INDUCED ASTHMA: THE MECHANISM

We mentioned in Chapter 2 that when we exercise, our lungs work more quickly than they do when we are walking or sitting. At the same time, the nasal passages have trouble purifying and warming all the additional air that enters the lungs as efficiently as they do under normal circumstances. The untreated air goes directly into the trachea and lungs. Air is treated even less when we breathe forcefully through the mouth. Very often air breathed through the mouth is drier and colder than air inhaled through the nose and causes our air passages to dry out and lose the moist blanket of mucus that normally protects them. As we pointed out earlier, people with asthma have very sensitive, or hyperreactive, air passages, so this untreated air is more likely to trigger an asthma flare.

Although they vary with each individual, symptoms of bronchoconstriction (which usually involve coughing or wheezing) usually appear five to ten minutes after beginning vigorous exercise. This timing can be affected by the weather. For example, if you run for ten minutes on a cold, dry day you will probably have more intense symptoms (and earlier into your run) than if you run on a day that is warm and humid.

EXERCISE: THE PHYSICAL BENEFITS

Although exercise is not a cure for asthma, it is a valuable part of asthma management. For a person with asthma, exercise has a number of physical benefits.

Cardiovascular Fitness

Through regular exercise, the heart and circulatory system can deliver increased amounts of oxygen to the entire body. This not only helps provide a reserve capacity of endurance when extra demands are placed on the body, it also helps lower cholesterol levels in the blood.

Exercise is especially important for asthma patients because good cardiovascular fitness will enable you to deal better with an asthma episode. It also will help you to recover your energy after one takes place. Through better cardiovascular fitness, you have something to fall back on during a difficult period.

Flexibility

Regular exercise is very important in helping you achieve a full range of body motion. Because physical exercise (especially yoga and calisthenics) causes you to move all your joints, it can help make the joints more flexible. This will give you the ability to use your body to the fullest, as it decreases the chance of pulling or straining muscles. When used in conjunction with deep breathing, regular exercise can also release tension in the chest, neck, and shoulders.

Endurance and Strength

We mentioned earlier that one of the side effects of long-term use of oral corticosteroids is muscle weakness. Exercise can reverse muscle weakness caused by these drugs. It can also build muscle endurance, and it permits you to enjoy more physical activities.

In addition, regular exercise can actually help reduce bronchial obstruction by improving mucus production and can lessen the frequency of asthma flares for both children and adults.

EXERCISE: THE PSYCHOLOGICAL BENEFITS

In addition to being good for your body, regular exercise is also good for your mind.

A Positive Mental Attitude

Regular exercise helps you develop self-esteem, optimism, and a "can do" attitude. This is especially important for asthma patients (and children in particular) who have always associated physical exertion with wheeziness, distress, discomfort, and defeat.

A Positive Self-Image

One of the most pleasant (and often unexpected) benefits of exercise is that it makes you look better. Exercise helps improve posture, clear the skin, and reduce excess body fat. This is especially important for children and others who take corticosteroids, because these steroids can stimulate the appetite and cause weight gain. Improved fitness and physique can help you feel better about yourself and more confident in social situations.

Finally, regular exercise helps you move away from the image of being sick and toward a positive self-image of attractiveness, health, and vitality.

WHICH EXERCISES ARE BEST?

Generally speaking, the best exercises for asthma patients are those that build strength, endurance, and flexibility. Aerobic exercises are especially recommended, because they increase the amount of oxygen in the blood and strengthen the heart and lungs. The most popular include running, dancing, swimming, and cycling. Because corticosteroids can decrease the strength of bones, your exercise regimen should involve a minimum of harsh pounding and joint trauma if you are taking steroids.

Fast walking; light, mild jogging; running on a treadmill; working out at a rowing machine; cycling (whether on the road or on a stationary cycle); Nautilus training; and low-impact aerobics are recommended for most asthma patients. The breathing and stretching involved in hatha-yoga exercises are also beneficial and safe for people with asthma, as are sports such as softball, volleyball, badminton, baseball, squash, water polo, golf, and tennis. Hiking is good, but sometimes pretreatment with a bronchodilator is recommended. This depends on the patient, the altitude, the time of the year, and how strenuous the hike is. Cross-country skiing is also recommended especially if you protect your mouth from cold air. Another recommended exercise for asthma patients is swimming, especially in warm water. The warm, moist environment of a heated pool provides adequate moisture to the lungs and decreases the risk of an asthma flare. Whether you swim laps or enjoy water aerobics, a warm pool can be an excellent place to exercise if you have asthma.

As we mentioned earlier, exercises that involve harsh pounding or joint trauma are generally not recommended for asthma patients. In addition to possibly damaging the brittle bones of people taking corticosteroids, severe jarring can sometimes trigger an asthma flare. Exercises that can involve jarring include contact sports such as football, rugby, soccer, and basketball. Bicycle racing (which often involves riding over bumpy roads at high speeds) and heavy jogging are included in this category. Running on a jogging machine may also be a problem, since some people who run on these devices can lose their balance and fall. Downhill skiers need to use extra caution to avoid falls while on the slopes. Jumping over moguls and hotdogging are not recommended for asthma patients on steroids and who also have brittle bones. While general weight training is beneficial to asthma patients, some exercise an-rehabilitation physical therapists feel that power lifting can be too stressful on the body. This doesn't mean that just because you have asthma you should automatically avoid these exercises. However, asthma patients—especially those who take oral steroids—should consult with their physician before doing them.

HOW MUCH EXERCISE?

Adults

Most physicians recommend at least forty minutes of exercise several times a week. This holds true for asthma patients as well, although forty minutes may be too much when you begin an exercise program. Ask your doctor or exercise therapist how you can build up your exercise level gradually and safely.

Children

Dr. Henry Milgram, a pediatrician at the National Jewish Center for Immunology and Respiratory Medicine, suggests that children with asthma should exercise thirty to forty minutes a day three or four times a week. He also advocates regular aerobics with adequate warm-up and cool-down before and after. Like adults, children should build up their exercise levels gradually, starting with sports or games that have built-in rest periods.

BEFORE EXERCISING: WHAT TO DO

1. Before beginning any exercise program, a complete fitness assessment is essential. It should be performed by a qualified professional under medical supervision. This assessment should include a treadmill test; an electrocardiogram; and muscle strength, flexibility, and lung capacity measurements. These tests will help your doctor determine if there are any other health problems that may limit the type and amount of exercise you can do.

   If you have exercise-induced bronchospasm, a measurement of peak flow is especially important, because it can give you a better idea of how you respond to different types of exercise. For example, a drop in peak flow is most marked when you run freely for ten to fifteen minutes, and is relatively small when you swim. All of these tests will enable your physician to help you create a well-rounded exercise program that will be both healthy and pleasurable.

2. Learn the fundamentals of efficient breathing, and take deep, slow, rhythmic breaths while exercising. People with asthma tend to hold their breath while exercising and should learn how to achieve regular, deep breathing during exercise periods. Of course, proper breathing is not only for asthma patients. Breathing instruction is a fundamental and accepted part of training in gymnastics, swimming, running, yoga, karate, and other physical activities. Unfortunately, it is often ignored in most school physical education classes.

3. Use medication as prescribed. Your physician may recommend that you take several puffs on a bronchodilator about ten minutes before beginning exercise. This has been found to be very helpful in preventing exercise-induced bronchospasm, both for children and adults. Bronchodi-

lators will also help relieve asthma symptoms once a flare has occurred. Cromolyn is not useful if taken during or after exercise, but is considered a good preventive medication. Because it can produce coughing, some patients take a bronchodilator before using cromolyn. Check with your doctor to see if this procedure is right for you.

4. Proper warm-up before exercise is essential. Long-distance runners do several short (ten-second) sprints before they begin running. This is to warm up the muscles gradually and prepare the body for the stress of exercise.

   If you like to run, you may want to begin by choosing activities that involve short sprints rather than sporting events calling for prolonged exercise, such as long-distance running. However, whatever exercise you choose, a cooling-down period is recommended after exercise is complete.

5. In winter, cold, dry air can trigger an asthma flare. For this reason, doctors recommend that you wear a face mask to breathe in warmer, moist air. It is also important to avoid strenuous exercise after a cold or during the pollen season. Infection or pollen may irritate your bronchial tubes and make it easier for exercise to bring on an asthma flare.

MODIFICATION: THE KEY

With the few exceptions mentioned above, you can enjoy almost any kind of sports activity. Unfortunately, many people have an "all or nothing" attitude about exercise: "If I can't run a mile, I won't run at all." If you are one of these people, *modification* is the key—especially when you begin an exercise program. Instead of playing nine holes of golf, you can play three. Bowl five frames at the lanes instead of ten. If cold air triggers asthma when you cycle outdoors, use an indoor exercise cycle. Instead of jogging outside, walk fast, or use a treadmill at the gym. Tennis does not need to be *competitive* tennis; it can be played for fun. Doubles tennis provides more opportunity for rest than singles tennis does.

Exercise and recreational therapists who work with asthma patients also stress the importance of starting an exercise program at a modest level and progressing gradually, increasing your level of activity by 10 percent or so a week. It is also good to pace yourself. For example, you can alternate between walking fast and walking slowly. You can also rest frequently during exercise rather than force yourself to do everything at once. As you gradually build up your strength and endurance, chances are good that you can eventually progress to normal levels of physical activity.

SEX AND ASTHMA

Although lovemaking is not exactly a sport, the same mechanism that causes exercise-induced asthma can take place during sexual activity. For many people with asthma, fear of an asthma attack while making love has put a damper on both their sex life and that of their partner. The greatest fear patients have is that the physical exertion involved during sex will trigger an attack or that kissing will be suffocating. Obviously, these fears do not contribute much to sexual desire!

The good news is that for the vast majority of asthma patients, a satisfying sex life is possible. However, preparation and modification are the keys to enjoyable sex for asthma patients and their partners, especially if asthma is moderate to severe.

As we mentioned earlier, regular aerobic-type exercise such as walking, swimming, or cycling builds endurance, strength, and flexibility. It also improves your physique and builds self-confidence. When you do any type of exercise, your breathing and heartbeat rates increase. They will also increase during lovemaking. However, since the amount of energy expended while making love is roughly equivalent to that of climbing a flight of stairs or taking a brisk walk, it should not pose difficulties for most asthma patients.

Physicians recommend that if your asthma is severe, you may want to use a bronchodilator ten to fifteen minutes before beginning sexual activity. You may also want to try less strenuous and more comfortable sexual positions during lovemaking. Making love with the partners lying on their sides, intercourse from a sitting position, or lovemaking with the asthma patient on top may make breathing easier for them. If you have severe asthma and require oxygen from time to time, it can easily be used in most lovemaking positions.

The old beliefs that sex is primarily a mechanical act that involves "performance" (especially on the part of the male) need to be discarded, both for the general public and for asthma patients in particular. Sex is essentially a creative expression of love and an intimate, sharing experience between lovers. It is not a sports event.

Finally, it is important that both partners communicate about how asthma may affect their sexual relationship. The partner should become aware of the patient's fears and concerns. For example, you can let your partner know which positions are most comfortable, or which activities make breathing easier for you. For some couples, lovemaking should be scheduled at those times of the day when the asthma patient feels best. While some people prefer sex to be more spontaneous, adapting to a more deliberate plan can create a special atmosphere of anticipation that can be very exciting for both of you.

If you are uncomfortable talking with your partner about your sexual relationship, consult your physician or other health professional. If they cannot help you, they may be able to refer you to someone who can. You may also want to obtain a copy of *Being Close,* an informative pamphlet about sex and respiratory disorders published by the National Jewish Center for Immunology and Respiratory Medicine. (See the Asthma Sources section for their address.)

Exercise-induced asthma is common among asthma patients, but it shouldn't limit your enjoyment of life. Giving up exercise is both unnecessary and harmful for both your mind and your body, and the benefits of regular exercise far outweigh the risks. By following the suggestions we've provided in this chapter, people with all but the severest asthma can enjoy regular, pleasurable physical activity without major limitations.

TEN

PSYCHOLOGICAL MANAGEMENT

Recent studies have found that on a psychological level, asthma patients are basically not different from other people. Like nonasthmatic individuals, some have conflicts with their mothers or their fathers. They have fears and insecurities. They have unresolved guilt feelings. The main difference is that they suffer from a chronic disease. It is mostly the disease itself that affects some of them psychologically rather than the other way around.

Not being able to breathe is one of the deepest of human fears. Living with asthma, which often involves unexpected, frightening, and debilitating symptoms, can be hellish. Panic, pain, and a genuine fear of dying are common, especially during severe attacks. A visit to an emergency room—particularly for a child—is often a traumatic experience that stays with the patient for years. For those who are affected by environmental trigger factors, the world can appear literally fraught with danger. Chronic problems with breathing often bring up feelings of insecurity, frustration, dependency, and helplessness. Anger and frustration are common among people with chronic disease, and asthma patients are no exception. Steroids can alter their physical appearance and make them feel unattractive and awkward. Many of the drugs used by asthma patients produce adverse side effects, which include mood swings, anxiety, and depression. Because these feelings are often directed toward family and friends, the asthma patient is sometimes branded as socially maladjusted.

It is important that people who are asthma-free have a better understanding of what an asthma patient goes through. It is also important for the asthma patient who is psychologically affected by the disease to know that his or her difficulties need not be permanent and that the way the patient deals with asthma psychologically can be improved through a variety of methods.

THE MAJOR PSYCHOLOGICAL ISSUES

A number of clinical studies have shown that both adults and children who suffer from serious asthma have more emotional and psychological problems than healthy people do. These problems are believed to be more as a *result* of having asthma rather than as a *cause* of asthma. However, as we have seen in Chapter 2, factors such as anxiety and depression also can play a role in triggering asthma.

The major problems (which are termed "poor coping mechanisms" by psychologists) include:

- negative self-image

- difficulty in adapting to new situations

- anger

- denial

- aggression

- fear of death or disability

- feelings of defeat

- depression

In addition, many children with severe asthma feel guilty for being a burden on the family. Because these emotions tend to be repressed, they are believed to play a role in making asthma flares worse. Finally, severity of illness, having another disease in addition to asthma, early (and multiple) visits to a hospital emergency room, and a chaotic or nonsupportive family environment tend to intensify psychological problems among children.

Vicious Circles

These psychological problems create *vicious circles* that can have a negative impact on your health. For example, feelings of anger or anxiety may cause hyperventilation and can trigger an asthma flare. This produces even greater upset and may make symptoms worse. It is also likely that the same vicious circle will be repeated periodically as long as you are unable to deal constructively with anger or anxiety.

"Benefits"

Another psychological issue involves the "benefits" of asthma. For example, if Johnny has an asthma flare when he gets angry, he discovers that his parents tend to discipline him less in order to avoid an asthma attack. Over a period of time he may be able to use asthma to avoid even the most minor parental discipline. Others can use asthma as a way to avoid taking an important test or fulfilling certain responsibilities; to get preferred treatment from teachers, parents, or peers; or to receive attention from others. Some patients depend on others (whether a parent, spouse, or doctor) for their care rather than take responsibility for their own health. If a particular person is meeting the patient's needs, there is no problem. But if the caretaker is not available, the patient becomes afraid or depressed. In many cases the patient's health can immediately deteriorate and may require emergency care.

Noncompliance

If an asthma sufferer is depressed over his or her condition, the patient may have a subconscious desire simply to give up. This may cause the patient to mislead the physician, disregard important symptoms, or fail to take correct doses of necessary medication. Noncompliance has been identified as a major cause of the growing number of emergency room visits and greatly increases the overall cost of medical care. It is also a component in the increasing death rate among asthma patients in general and adolescents in particular.

These problems are relatively common among persons with chronic illnesses and should be addressed and dealt with by both the patient and the physician. It is important to deal with these major life issues and resolve them before effective self care for asthma can begin. Let's briefly explore some of the major ways that can lead to that goal: education, preventive strategies, ongoing counseling, relaxation, hypnosis, biofeedback, and psychological support.

EDUCATION

If you are an asthma patient, you need to discuss your expectations about care as well as understand your physician's goals. The doctor should also discuss the benefits of the medications prescribed, as well as their side effects. He or she also needs to provide you with the knowledge and skills needed to take medication properly and to handle treatments or procedures necessary for proper self-care. You also should learn about diet, exercise, ways to measure peak flow, and recognize the need for emergency care. When patients have a clear understanding of their asthma and their role in managing it, they tend to feel more in control of their lives. This understanding increases self-esteem, engenders positive feelings about treatment, and strengthens the belief that asthma can indeed be controlled. Greater patient responsibility and improved doctor-patient cooperation naturally follow.

PREVENTIVE STRATEGIES

Once asthma has been diagnosed, the factors that trigger asthma should be determined as soon as possible. The second step is to do what's necessary to limit those trigger factors. This includes establishing a hypoallergenic home environment, paying attention to diet, learning proper exercise techniques, and taking periodic peak-flow readings. It also means knowing what medications to take and how to administer them properly. These strategies can limit the number of severe asthma symptoms and multiple emergency hospitalizations, which often prove to be stressful for asthma patients and their families.

ONGOING COUNSELING

You and your doctor must work as a team to manage asthma. It is important that you feel comfortable consulting with your physician about any problems regarding asthma symptoms and triggers, any changes in the course of your treatment, and any side effects from medication. The doctor also should be aware of depression, anxiety, or problems with compliance on the part of the patient. For most patients, just being able to share their feelings, questions, and concerns with the physician is all they need to maintain normal functioning. If more serious problems exist, whether on physical or emotional levels, your physician may want to refer you to a specialist.

RELAXATION

Learning how to relax is an important part of managing your asthma. Good relaxation techniques make you more aware of specific factors that trigger anxiety and teach you how to deal with them in a constructive way. For some people, relaxation may simply involve learning how to communicate their needs and feelings to family members and friends rather than keeping those feelings repressed. For others, relaxation may involve learning not to hook into a particular issue that may trigger a stressful reaction.

Specific relaxation techniques can also help. They often include deep breathing and positive mental imagery, which can help the patient achieve a calm, relaxed state of mind. Dr. Ainslie Meares, an Australian psychiatrist, wrote in *Relief Without Drugs* (Fontana-Collins, 1967) that mental relaxation exercises are vital for every asthma patient and can help reduce both the frequency and severity of attacks in at least two out of three. Because relaxation can also help reduce the need for medication, he suggested that patients work with their physician over a period of time to adjust medication as needed. There are many books that can teach you how to relax, and classes in stress-reduction are sometimes taught in health clubs and adult education schools. Some organizations—both spiritually oriented and not—offer classes in meditation. Your physician may also be able to recommend someone who teaches relaxation methods in your community. However, remember that relaxation techniques are not a quick fix for asthma and that they usually work best when practiced regularly over weeks or months.

HYPNOSIS

Hypnosis has sometimes been useful to asthma patients. For some individuals, changes in the air passages can be induced by suggestion. Studies in Great Britain revealed that when asthma patients are told that they are being given a bronchodilator, for example, the airways will expand even if the substance is inert. Hypnosis may also be able to help some patients deal more constructively with anxiety by altering traditional response patterns to stress. Some individuals respond better to hypnosis than others do, so rates of success vary considerably. It is also important to remember that hypnosis should only be performed by a qualified professional, such as a licensed psychologist or psychiatrist.

BIOFEEDBACK

Biofeedback is a training program designed to help the individual control involuntary body functions such as heartbeat, blood pressure, muscle tension, and skin temperature. Using special monitoring devices that measure, for example, changes in blood pressure, brain waves, and muscle contractions, the patient learns how to reproduce desired changes through breathing, relaxation, and positive mental imagery. Biofeedback has been used by asthma patients to help reduce anxiety and to open up the breathing passages. Like hypnosis, biofeedback studies with asthma patients of all ages have shown varied results. However, since it can cause no harm to asthma patients, many feel that biofeedback may be worth a try. For the name of a qualified biofeedback practitioner in your area, contact the Biofeedback Certification Institute of America (see the Asthma Sources section).

PSYCHOLOGICAL SUPPORT

Living with a chronic disease such as asthma isn't easy. Long-term illness often erodes self-confidence and can engender anger and fear. These feelings can and often do affect our work, family life, and other relationships. Psychological support is very important for people with asthma. You may want to vent your feelings or concerns periodically with a friend or relative. You may prefer to consult with your physician or clergy-member, or a social worker, therapist, or other professional. The type of support you choose depends not just on the issues involved but also on your goals and needs as well.

Psychotherapy

Psychotherapy is a very broad term that encompasses suggestion, reeducation, psychoanalysis, and other forms of therapy such as bioenergetics. Psychotherapy can benefit the asthma patient in two basic ways. First, it can help you cope with the stresses of normal living that may play a role in triggering asthma in the first place. Difficulties in relationships, problems at work or at school, or poor adaptation to life's challenges are among the most common of these stresses.

Psychotherapy can also help you to cope better with your disease and deal with the emotional problems that asthma may cause. These problems may include anxiety, anger, fear, denial, and depression. Therapy can also provide insights into areas of concern such as self-esteem, communication, and proper self-care.

For some patients who suffer from depression, antidepressant drugs may be indicated. They should be prescribed only after a thorough medical and psychological evaluation and should not interfere with any other medications the patient may be taking for asthma or other diseases.

Family Counseling

Some people have said that when one family member has asthma, the whole family has asthma. Like other chronic diseases, asthma can be very disruptive to normal family life. If the patient is a child, he or she may take the lion's share of attention from the parents. The other children may be resentful. Asthma can also be a drain on the family's income and can disrupt vacation and recreation time. Anger, guilt, and depression may affect interaction among family members.

Family counseling can be helpful in dealing with these issues. Counseling will vary according to the particular needs of the family. In some cases, family members will be educated about asthma and how it can be controlled. They can also be given a greater understanding of what the asthma patient has to deal with. Negative feelings can be explored in a safe atmosphere. Creative solutions can be found to everyday problems that pose difficulty. Persons with asthma tend to do better if they perceive a support network around them, and tend to do poorly if they feel that the family unit is chaotic and nonsupportive.

Group Therapy

Group therapy can provide educational, therapeutic, and social support for people with asthma. Therapy and discussion groups offer a supportive environment where patients can share problems, concerns, and fears with others. Groups also provide patients with peer models who are successfully dealing with asthma in their lives. Some physicians, hospitals, and local lung associations sponsor discussion groups for asthma patients. They are often free or are low in cost. It is sometimes difficult to become involved with a group of "strangers," but after a few minutes in the group, these feelings usually disappear. Being with people who are dealing with the same issues as you are can be a very supportive experience.

Although dealing with a chronic disease such as asthma is often difficult and frustrating, it can also help you grow emotionally. By learning how to deal with the psychological issues of asthma you can become more self-aware, enjoy greater insights about yourself and your relationships, and better decide what is really important in your life. For some, asthma has even been a motivation for self-transformation. By cultivating a positive attitude about life and trying to view every challenge as an opportunity, your relationship with a disease such as asthma can change. As you learn how to cope with a difficult situation, you can also use asthma as a tool to develop positive human qualities such as self-awareness, patience, compassion, and understanding.

Art Therapy

Art therapy has proven successful with young asthma patients, although it can benefit people of all ages. It gives them a chance to vent their feelings of anger and fear. By learning from the clues that drawings and paintings provide, the therapist can assess patients' relationships to other members of the family as well as how they view themselves and their disease. Art therapy is effective because, in part, it gives people suffering from asthma the opportunity to disassociate themselves from their disease. As a result, they are freer in expressing often repressed feelings and attitudes. It has been found to be very effective in helping children improve coping skills.

ELEVEN

COMPLEMENTARY THERAPIES

So far we've talked about mainstream medical therapies. Bu
many people report that certain nontraditional therapies may
also be helpful in controlling asthma.

There are at least 130 different systems for treating human
ailments. They include ancient therapies from the East such as
ayurveda and acupuncture as well as more recent Western
developments such as chiropractic and homeopathy. Tradi
tional Western medicine (known as "allopathic medicine") is
one of these systems of curing disease. It is based on the idea
that in order to treat a disease symptom, a medicine or proce
dure should be used to produce effects different from the
symptom. For example, if your airways are narrowed, a medi
cation is given to open them up. If you have a fever, a cold
compress is given to cool you off. Allopathy is by far the domi
nant health-care system in this country and most other West
ern industrialized nations.

The treatments of allopathic medicine are based on exhaus
tive clinical trials that can take many years. New medications
are tested on hundreds of patients, using a placebo to help
verify the effectiveness of a specific medication or therapeutic
procedure. These studies are often funded by the government

drug companies, and private foundations. In contrast, evidence that supports the effectiveness of other forms of health care are often based on anecdotes, informal surveys, and individual success stories. Because they are not part of the medical mainstream, practitioners of health care systems such as homeopathy, herbal medicine, and chiropractic do not enjoy the prestige or the funding that traditional physicians do.

In the United States and Canada, traditional medical therapy is seen as the treatment of choice for asthma. Many physicians feel that the hope of finding an effective medication or treatment outside of the medical mainstream is a waste of time and effort. They also warn that seeking out other therapies is a form of noncompliance, and using alternative therapies can be downright dangerous when the asthma is severe or chronic. In Europe, however, allopathic medicine is not viewed as the only way to treat asthma. In Great Britain, for example, where asthma research is considered by some to be several years ahead of that in the United States, the medical community is far more open to other health care modalities such as homeopathic medicine when it comes to asthma prevention and treatment.

This doesn't mean that if you're taking theophylline several times a day you should give up your medication and try herbal teas instead. Until we know for certain that an alternative treatment is better than one that has already been scientifically proven, replacing a proven medication with something else can be risky, especially when asthma is severe or difficult to manage. For this reason we suggest that the treatments described on the following pages be considered *for information only* and be viewed as possible *complementary* therapies rather than as alternatives to traditional medical care. Most can be used while continuing your present course of medical therapy, although some—such as herbs and Chinese medicine—involve specific doses that may cause side effects or interfere with regular medical treatment.

The complementary therapies discussed on the following pages are explored only briefly. If any appeal to you, find out more about them in your local library or bookstore. The better educated you are as a patient, the wiser, more informed choices you will make regarding your health care. Finally, the importance of working as a team with your physician in managing asthma cannot be underestimated. When considering other types of health care methods for dealing with asthma, consult with your physician before changing your present course of treatment in any way.

ACUPUNCTURE AND ACUPRESSURE

The ancient Chinese system of *acupuncture* has been around for thousands of years, but was ignored by Western physicians until the 1970s, when it was found to aid in anesthesia before surgery. As it became more accepted in this country and in Europe, patients have testified to its success in strengthening the immune system and in treating a wide variety of diseases, including high blood pressure, ulcer, migraine headaches, asthma, and heart disease. Among nonallopathic methods, acupuncture is the most accepted form of asthma treatment in the West.

The Goal

The major goal of acupuncture is to treat disease by regulating the functioning of the entire organism. It seeks to strengthen or reinforce organs of the body that are deficient, and it drains or sedates areas that are functioning in excess. Diagnosis involves examining the patient's back by touching (palpating) certain areas to determine places that are tense or sensitive.

Procedure

After a careful and thorough diagnosis, the practitioner works to stimulate the flow of life energy (known as *ch'i*) to poorly functioning organs by puncturing certain points of the body with special needles. These points (known as *pinyin*) number eight hundred to one thousand and are divided into twelve main groups. All the points in each group are united by a line called a *meridian*, of which there are fourteen. Each acupuncture point has both a Chinese name and a number and is related to a specific organ. For example, the *taiyuan* point, or "L-9," is related to the lungs. The points stimulated may involve other organs as well as the organ in question. For example, panting and wheezing symptoms associated with asthma are also associated with the lungs, spleen, and kidneys. It is believed that when these points are blocked, the *ch'i* is unable to descend. When performed with skill and exactitude, the treatments are rarely painful, and infection from needles is uncommon. By inserting the needles into specific points at prescribed angles for differing lengths of time (usually no more than several minutes), the acupuncturist is able to induce feelings of stimulation, numbness, swelling, or a sense of heaviness in certain parts of the body that are linked to the meridian being treated.

Although not well understood by Western scientists, it is believed that acupuncture may block certain impulses from the spinal cord, thus affecting nerve transmission to affected parts of the body. Others believe that acupuncture can affect the human energy field, which in turn can affect the function of body cells.

In the treatment of asthma there are a number of points routinely used by acupuncturists. They include the *dingchuan* (M-BW-1), *tiantu* (CO-22), *xuanji* (CO-21), and *shanzhong* (CO-17). Five supplementary points are also used, both alone and in combination with others. In the case of severe asthma, for example, a total of ten points are used. Acupuncture is used both during and between asthma attacks. Although there are no medical studies regarding acupuncture and asthma published in the West, some patients report a decrease in both the frequency and severity of attacks. Some have also been able to reduce their asthma medication through regular acupuncture treatments.

Professional Qualifications

The professional qualifications of acupuncturists vary considerably. Some, including medical doctors and chiropractors, may have taken a short course in the basics of acupuncture and can legally practice it as an adjunct to their primary profession. Other acupuncturists have taken an exhaustive study and training course that can last several years or more in a recognized institution in the United States or China. Some states license acupuncturists; others do not.

Acupuncture is considered among the safest health care modalities. However, when choosing a practitioner of acupuncture or any health care system, know their qualifications and experience before placing yourself in their care.

ACUPRESSURE

Acupressure (known as *shiatsu* in Japan) is closely related to acupuncture but involves applying firm pressure of the fingertips to specific contact points (of which there are 102) throughout the body rather than puncturing them with needles. Since acupressure is somewhat less specific than acupuncture, acupressure is not considered to be as effective in the management of asthma. However, the main advantages to acupressure are that it does not involve puncturing the skin, and it can be performed at home by a trained family member. Acupressure texts describe six specific points on the back that can reduce asthma symptoms, as well as three above the rib cage and two on the arm.

Professional Qualifications

As is the case regarding the practice of acupuncture, individual states have different laws regulating the training and practice of acupressure therapists. In some states they need to have graduated from an accredited school of acupressure and be certified by a state board of licensure. In others they merely need to put up a shingle.

CHIROPRACTIC

Chiropractic deals with the vital relationship between the nervous system and the spinal column, and the role of this relationship in the restoration and maintenance of health. Chiropractic was developed in the United States nearly a hundred years ago by Daniel David Palmer and has become the largest drugless health-care method in the Western world.

The Goal

The philosophy of chiropractic teaches that our ability to adapt to changes in our internal and external environments is essential to good health. This ability depends on an unobstructed flow of nerve impulses from the brain through the spinal nerves and onward to every cell of the body, thus guiding their every function. There is a return flow as well. Every part of the body is constantly sending messages regarding its function and environment back to the brain. The brain responds appropriately in a fraction of a second to maintain the organ or tissue in good condition.

Chiropractic teaches that when vertebrae of the spinal column become misaligned or *subluxated,* they can impinge on delicate spinal nerves and interfere with the proper flow of nerve impulses between the brain and the organs, tissues, and cells of the body. Chiropractors believe that this obstruction can eventually impair the body's ability to stay healthy and can lay the groundwork for actual disease symptoms, including those of asthma.

Procedure

The chiropractor (known as a D.C. or Doctor of Chiropractic) must locate and adjust the subluxated vertebrae so that nerve interference can be removed. He or she first examines the spine to determine which bones are out of alignment. Hands may be used to palpate the spine, or heat-sensitive instruments or X rays may be used instead. When the chiropractor determines which bones are out of alignment, painless corrective adjustments are made to realign the vertebrae and reduce pressure on spinal nerves. When the body's organs and tissues receive an unobstructed nerve supply from the brain, chiropractors believe that the body will return to a state of health and protect itself from illness. Because it is the body that heals itself, most chiropractors do not claim to treat disease, including asthma.

Professional Qualifications

Unlike practitioners of other alternative systems, all chiropractors must be duly licensed by the state in which they practice, and all must be graduates of a federally accredited chiropractic college. Only licensed chiropractors (they will always have D.C. after their name) are qualified to perform specialized chiropractic adjustments.

Until recently the American Medical Association barred medical doctors from referring patients to chiropractors or working with them in any way. Since a landmark antitrust decision against the AMA in 1987, there has been greater communication and cooperation between members of the two professions. Some chiropractors and medical doctors even have joint practices.

The ability of chiropractic in relieving the frequency and intensity of asthma is disputed by members of the medical profession. David A. Mrazek, M.D., of the National Jewish Center for Immunology and Respiratory Medicine suggests that it is easy to speculate that a treatment is effective, but scientific evidence is needed before we put our faith in it. He points out that there is no scientific evidence that proves that chiropractic cures asthma, and advises that until such evidence is forthcoming, patients should be cautious about using chiropractic to cure it. Other physicians cite cases where chiropractic made the asthma patient delay seeking needed medical care or discontinue taking essential medication.

While chiropractors do not guarantee an asthma cure, they claim that chiropractic adjustments have been of tremendous benefit to patients with asthma. They point out that the medical doctor sees only the chiropractic failures and that many asthma patients have come to chiropractors only after medical science had failed them.

OSTEOPATHIC MEDICINE

Modern osteopathy is now a small element within the medical mainstream. In addition to traditional medical therapy, an osteopath (known as a Doctor of Osteopathy or a D.O.) may also manipulate bones, muscles, and connective tissue (fascia) to help your body fight disease. Although most osteopathic physicians prescribe traditional allopathic drugs to control asthma, some practitioners believe that breathing primarily with the chest muscles (and through the mouth) can overstimulate the sympathetic nervous system and contribute to an asthma attack. By using gentle manipulation, osteopaths help restore abdominal breathing. They also encourage you to breathe through the nose and teach you stress reduction techniques to help prevent asthma flares.

HOMEOPATHIC MEDICINE

Homeopathy was developed nearly two hundred years ago, in Philadelphia, by German physician Samuel Christian Heinemann. It was a respected form of medical treatment in the United States until only the turn of the century, but continues to enjoy wide prestige in Europe. There are six homeopathic hospitals in Britain, and the Royal Family uses homeopathy as their health-care system of choice.

The Goal

Unlike allopathic medicine, which treats disease by using drugs that produce actions different from the symptoms being treated (such as a bronchodilator to open up narrowed air passages or a decongestant to dry up mucus), homeopathy teaches that the body gets rid of disease through symptoms. Therefore, homeopaths prescribe substances that elicit in healthy people symptoms similar to those of the disease.

Procedure

The homeopathic physician takes a very long and detailed history of the patient that encompasses not only symptoms but also life-style, diet, and personality. Homeopaths generally spend a great deal of time getting to know the patient rather than focusing on objective symptoms only. Homeopathic medicine uses only natural preparations made from animal, vegetable, or mineral sources. They are nontoxic, nonhabit-forming, and cause no side effects.

Depending on the factors that contribute to the attack, asthma patients have used such substances as ipecacuana, carbo vegetabilis, arsenicum album, and nux vomica.

Professional Qualifications

In the United States a homeopath must also be a licensed allopathic practitioner (M.D.).

To derive maximum benefit from homeopathic remedies for asthma, they should be taken only after consultation with a homeopathic physician.

HERBAL MEDICINE

Herbs have been used to treat human ailments since prehistoric times. Herbal remedies are referred to in the Bible and can be found in Chinese herbals dating to 2700 B.C. Although herbs are often viewed as alternative medicine, many orthodox medications, including asthma drugs such as cromolyn, beta agonists, and theophylline, are derived from plant sources.

Please keep in mind that we are not recommending herbal therapy for asthma. It is difficult to find a qualified herbalist, and it is certainly unwise to attempt self-treatment. Nonetheless, some asthma patients report that herbal remedies have relieved their symptoms, so we are including an overview of herbal medicine for information only.

The Goal

The idea behind herbal medicine is to stimulate the body's own defenses rather than treat symptoms only. Because herbal doses are relatively small, the chances for adverse side effects are remote. Herbal remedies can be made either from the leaf, bark, fruit, stem, or root of the plant. They are usually consumed as a tea (infusion), although some are made into a poultice, powder, juice, or vapor bath.

A wide variety of herbs are reputed to manage asthma. Some are used by themselves or in combination with other herbs. In Western herbology they include celedine, coltsfoot, horehound, lobelia, skunk cabbage, thyme (as a bath), valerian, and yerba santa. In Chinese herbal medicine, Chinese wolfberry, boxthorn, sweet almond, ginseng, and licorice are common. However, the botanical of choice is ephedra, which has been used in China since the second century. It is contained in a prepared medication called *chih ke pien*. Chinese herbalists also mix datura metel with tobacco and smoke them together in a cigarette. Some Chinese herbs used in asthma treatment, such as bitter almond, have toxic effects and should be used with caution.

Although many herbs can be found in natural-food stores

and herb shops (especially in larger cities), it is best to consult a trained professional herbalist before you decide to experiment with a particular herbal remedy. A good herbalist will not only discuss your symptoms with you but also will evaluate your diet, life-style, and health history. Herbalists are aware of other substances (some of which may cause interactions with medication) that the herb they prescribe may contain.

Professional Qualifications

Since herbalism is a relatively new profession in this country, it is more difficult finding a qualified herbalist in the United States than it is in many European countries, where they are certified and licensed. However, many good practitioners have earned a degree as a Naturopathic Physician (N.D.) from a licensed school of naturopathy in the United States or Europe. In addition, many acupuncturists receive instruction in prescribing Chinese herbs for asthma and other diseases.

While acknowledging that herbs can play in role in asthma management, some orthodox physicians express reservations. They point out that many patients are only told of the benefits of a particular herb without being made aware of possible dangers. They also say that the doses given are often in inexact amounts. Some prepared herbal medications may also contain a steroid or other substance that may not be beneficial to the patient, while others may be nothing more than fly-by-night remedies that are of little value. Finally, traditional medical doctors point out that the drugs they give for asthma contain only the isolated medication that may be found in the herb, while the herbs in their natural state may contain other substances. In contrast, herbalists believe that these secondary substances may well make the primary substance safer and more effective.

YOGA

The ancient Indian science of yoga has been found to benefit some asthma patients. The mental and physical effects of stretching, deep breathing, and mind-quieting techniques that are part of yoga practice may have a calming effect that can reduce the frequency and severity of asthma flares.

In an Indian study of 106 asthma patients reported in the *British Medical Journal,* half of the participants were asked to perform an integrated series of yoga exercises including deep breathing, breath-slowing techniques, meditation, and a devotional session for 65 minutes a day for two weeks. The remaining 53 patients with comparable symptoms continued taking only their normal asthma medications. By the end of the study the group that practiced yoga showed improved peak-flow rates and fewer asthma flares, and required less medication than the other group.

Other studies have shown that yogic breathing, stretching, and meditation can lower the metabolic rate and can stabilize and reduce the excitability of the nervous system. Because yoga has also been found to reduce the activity of the vagus nerve (which has been recognized as playing a role in regulating bronchoconstriction), it is effective in helping asthma patients have fewer and less severe asthma episodes.

One of the advantages to yoga is that it can be easily practiced at home by people of all ages. You can find a number of fine study courses in your local library or bookstore. Yoga classes are also offered in yoga centers, health clubs, and adult education classes in many communities.

On the preceding pages we've examined the major complementary therapies that have been found to be useful to some asthma patients. However, you may want to explore reflexology, therapeutic touch, visualization, and ayurvedic medicine as well.

TWELVE

THE FUTURE OF ASTHMA MANAGEMENT

As we have seen on the preceding pages, asthma is a very complex disease that can involve a wide variety of trigger factors. Asthma has been a serious medical challenge for centuries, and it is likely to continue being a serious challenge in the future. Although new medications and improved monitoring systems have been developed to prevent and control asthma in recent years, there is still much to do. Many people—especially asthma patients and their families—wonder what may be in store in the future. Let's look at some of the new trends.

MEDICATIONS

Medical science will continue to discover and develop effective remedies that will help prevent and manage asthma attacks. At the time of this writing, over seventy asthma medications are under review for approval by the U.S. Food and Drug Administration (FDA). Dozens more are being developed. Some have to do with controlling hyperactivity of the airways, preventing exercise-induced asthma, and managing nighttime asthma attacks. Other drugs have been developed to inhibit the synthesis or the release of mediators (chemicals released by the mast cell that trigger an asthma attack). Several others are being designed to work with specific trigger factors, such as sulfur dioxide or cold air.

Among these medications, a number of drugs are being developed (or are awaiting FDA approval) that will have fewer side effects than some commonly used medications such as theophylline. One such medication is enprofyline, which is, like theophylline, a methylxanthine bronchodilator. Among adrenergic bronchodilators, fenoterol and procaterol are pending approval by the FDA. Some nonbronchodilator drugs designed to prevent asthma attacks include lodoxamide, ketotifen, and azelastine. Ketotifen has already been approved in Europe. In addition to preventing the occurrence of asthma symptoms, azelastine may have a bronchodilator effect as well. Because researchers believe it to have a minimum of adverse side effects, ketotifen is being considered as a possible alternative to theophylline.

Other therapies now being explored include gamma globulin therapy to help restore balance in the immune system, and taking extra vitamin B_6 (pyridoxine). It is believed that this vitamin may inhibit the development of a certain chemical (serotonin) found in the mast cell and thus reduce the likelihood of an asthma flare.

GETTING AT THE GENETIC CAUSE

We've pointed out earlier that asthma is primarily an inherited disease. Some researchers believe that a major effort toward finding an asthma cure involves unraveling the genetic code so they can identify the specific gene associated with asthma. Researchers in England have recently come upon the abnormality of a single gene that they have traced to chromosome 11. By understanding the gene's exact function, doctors are hopeful that they will be able to devise new methods of prevention and treatment.

HOLISM

Another major development in medical care that will become more important in helping asthma patients in the future is a holistic approach to health care. Because holistic health is a relatively new term to many, it is often misunderstood. Let's briefly examine what it is and how it will be helpful to the asthma patient.

Holism acknowledges the fundamental wholeness and unity of the individual and how we interact with the environment. As a patient, we are viewed as an open system rather than as a collection of airtight compartments, such as "heart," "airways," and "emotions." Holistic health care addresses our attitudes, emotions, relationships, family situation, diet, exercise, and other life-style patterns as well as specific disease symptoms. Some holistic practitioners also explore spiritual aspects of health, an idea almost totally absent from orthodox medicine.

The National Jewish Center for Immunology and Respiratory Medicine in Denver was the first major institution in the country to put this comprehensive approach to asthma care (with the exception of the spiritual aspect just mentioned) into practice. Its residency program has the patient working with a team of medical doctors, psychologists, physical and recreation therapists, and dietitians. The staff not only helps to educate the patient about the dynamics of asthma, what drugs to take, and how to identify and reduce exposure to trigger factors, but also examines the patient's family dynamics, how the family deals with stress, and how a good diet and proper exercise can help manage the disease. The patient is considered as a total, integrated unit rather than as merely a collection of symptoms.

"Holistic" versus "Alternative"

Holistic health care is often confused with alternative or complementary therapies, although they are very different. For example, by itself herbal medicine is not holistic. When a herbalist gives you a herbal preparation to open up your bronchial tubes, he or she is not necessarily dealing with you as a whole person: the practitioner is treating your physical symptoms. This approach, like that of traditional medicine, is dualistic and reductionistic: it is dealing with a physical problem (bronchospasm) by stimulating or inhibiting the functions of the airways. However, if a herbalist is also concerned about your diet, emotions, and life-style and how they impact on the health problem, the practitioner is taking a more holistic approach to health. As we begin to see the value of a well rounded approach to health care, more holistic approaches to asthma care will be adopted among even the most conservative of practitioners.

Nobody wants to experience a chronic illness, and asthma is among the most unpleasant. However, asthma is one disease that can be effectively managed by the vast majority of asthma sufferers. To do so requires knowledge, patience, and awareness of one's outer and inner environments. By understanding asthma and how it affects you, you begin to take charge of your life. In working as a partner with your physician to prevent and manage asthma symptoms, you begin to claim your true inner power. Through this combination of self-awareness, practical knowledge, and self-empowerment you can learn how to achieve your fullest health potential, both in the present and in the future.

GLOSSARY

adrenaline A hormone produced by the sympathetic nervous system that can, among other things, relax bronchial tubes. Also known as epinephrine.

allergen Any substance that brings on symptoms of allergy.

allergy An altered reaction of body tissues to a specific substance (allergen) that will not produce a reaction in nonallergic individuals.

alveoli Minute air sacs in the lungs. This is where oxygen and carbon dioxide are exchanged between the blood and the air.

anaphylaxis An extreme adverse reaction to a foreign substance such as an allergen, food, or drug.

antibody A protein substance produced by the immune system in response to an antigen.

antigen A bacteria, toxin, or foreign blood cell that is capable of stimulating an immune response, such as the production of antibodies.

antihistamine A drug that blocks the effect of histamine on the body.

arterial blood gases A lab test designed to measure the amount of oxygen and carbon dioxide in the blood.

atopic asthma Asthma due to inherited allergy.

autonomic nervous system The part of the nervous system that is connected with the control of involuntary body functions such as breathing, heartbeat, and glandular activity.

beta blockers Drugs (usually used for high blood pressure and heart disorders) that produce constriction of the bronchioles as a side effect. They are usually harmful for asthma patients.

beta-2 agonists Drugs that act on receptors to relax bronchial muscles.

bronchi Air passages through which air moves to and from the lungs. Also known as bronchial tubes.

bronchioles Small air passages that branch off from the bronchi.

bronchitis Inflammation of the bronchial tubes.

bronchoconstriction Narrowing of the air passages.

bronchodilator A drug used to open up the air passages. Bronchodilators can be used for both the prevention and the treatment of asthma symptoms.

bronchospasm Narrowing of the air passages due to a sudden tightening of the bronchial muscles.

carbon dioxide The gas that humans and other animals breathe out. It's produced as a normal part of body metabolism.

cilia Tiny wavy hairs that are designed to remove mucus, germs, pollen, and dust from the air passages.

corticosteroids Drugs that are similar to hormones produced by the cortex of the adrenal gland. They are often used to reduce inflammation of the bronchial passages.

cromolyn A drug used to stabilize mast cells and thus help prevent asthma symptoms.

cyanosis A blue tinge of the nails, lips, and skin caused by deficiencies of oxygen and an excess of carbon dioxide in the blood. It sometimes occurs during a severe asthma flare.

dander Skin scurf or dandruff.

diaphragm A muscle between the lungs and the stomach. It is used especially when we breathe deeply.

dilation Expansion or opening of a vessel or organ such as the air passages.

dyspnea Air hunger resulting in labored or difficult breathing. It often occurs in moderate to severe asthma flares.

edema Swelling of body tissues due to an excessive amount of fluid.

emphysema A chronic airways disease that affects the alveoli and makes them less resilient.

epinephrine See *adrenaline*.

extrinsic asthma Asthma triggered by exposure to an allergen.

FEV_1 The amount of air forcibly exhaled in one second.

histamine A common mediator linked to asthma.

hyperreactive airways Airways that overreact to a stimulus. This often involves tightening or narrowing.

hyperventilation Increased inspiration and expiration caused by deeper and/or faster breathing. It can produce anxiety, low blood pressure, and dizziness.

immune response The body's natural reaction to foreign substances.

immunoglobulin E (IgE) A particular type of antibody. In patients with asthma, an excess of IgE causes mediators to be released that produce an allergic reaction.

immunotherapy A form of medical treatment designed to reduce a person's sensitivity to a particular substance. This may include allergy shots.

inhaler An aerosol device used to administer medication to a patient's lungs while the patient breathes in.

intrinsic asthma Asthma in which allergy does not play a large part. It is often associated with other respiratory problems, such as bronchitis.

mast cells Large cells located throughout the body, including the bronchial tubes, and that release substances (such as histamine) under certain circumstances.

mediator A chemical released by mast cells to protect the body from allergens.

metered dose inhaler See **inhaler**.

mucus A sticky liquid that coats the air passages. It traps most of the germs, pollen, and dust that we breathe in.

nebulizer An apparatus used by asthma patients that delivers medication through the mouth as a fine mist or spray. It is more powerful than a metered dose inhaler.

peak expiratory flow rate The maximum rate at which air can be exhaled. Measured in liters per second.

peak-flow meter A device used to measure peak expiratory flow. A drop in normal flow indicates a possible asthma flare.

pulmonary function tests Tests given to see how well the lungs are functioning.

radioallergosorbent test (RAST) A test designed to measure IgE in the blood.

receptor Molecular group in cells that have a special affinity for allergens or toxins.

skin test A test for allergy done by either scratching or lightly puncturing the skin and exposing the surface to a suspected allergen.

smooth muscles Muscles (such as those surrounding the air passages) over which we have no direct control.

spacer An apparatus inserted between an inhaler and the patient's mouth to increase the amount of medication reaching the lungs.

spasm A sudden involuntary tightening of the muscles.

spirometer An apparatus used to measure air volume in the lungs.

sputum Dirty mucus and other material brought up from the lungs.

status asthmaticus   Severe asthma that is persistent and very difficult to control.

steroids   A group of hormones naturally produced by the body that share a similar chemical makeup. Synthesized steroids are used as asthma medications to help prevent asthma flares.

theophylline   A popular bronchodilator that is chemically related to caffeine.

trachea   The windpipe.

triggers   Substances (such as pollen) or conditions (such as exercise) that can set off an asthma flare.

ventilation   Medical term for breathing.

wheezing   A hissing or whistling sound caused by difficulty breathing.

SOURCES

American Lung Association
1740 Broadway
New York, N.Y. 10019
   Provides educational information about asthma and other lung diseases. It can also suggest summer camps for children with asthma. Branches in every state.

Asthma Society of Canada
P.O. Box 213
Station K
Toronto, Ont. M4P 2G5
   Provides educational information about asthma.

Asthma Society, and Friends of the
   Asthma Research Council
300 Upper Street
London N1 2XX England
   The Asthma Society is the primary resource for asthma education and information in Great Britain. The group offers a variety of pamphlets and publishes *Asthma News,* a monthly newsletter.

Asthmatic Children's Foundation
15 Spring Valley Road
Ossining, N.Y. 10562

Provides treatment and rehabilitation for children with severe asthma. Also provides educational materials and publishes the *Journal of Asthma*.

Biofeedback Certification Institute of America
10200 West 44th Avenue
Wheat Ridge, Colo. 80033

This organization provides certification for all biofeedback practitioners in the United States.

Mothers of Asthmatics, Inc.
10875 Main Street, Suite 210
Fairfax, Va. 22030

This organization provides support for parents of children with asthma. Publishes an annual resource list including names of camps and equipment vendors, as well as a regular newsletter, the *MA Report*.

The National Foundation for Asthma, Inc.
P.O. Box 30069
Tucson, Ariz. 85751

Provides health services for asthma patients, especially those with financial hardship.

National Heart, Lung, and Blood Institute
NIH Building 31, Room 4A-21
9000 Rockville Pike
Bethesda, Md. 20892

This institute provides a free listing of asthma publications and resources, and has produced several educational programs for asthma patients and their families.

National Jewish Center for Immunology
  and Respiratory Medicine
1400 Jackson Street
Denver, Colo. 80206
(800) 222-LUNG; (303) 355-LUNG (within Colorado)

This is the leading medical institute for treating asthma and other lung diseases, and is recommended for those who are suffering from chronic, severe asthma that is not improving with present medical care. In addition to offering an innovative multidisciplinary treatment program that is recognized worldwide, National Jewish offers a variety of free publications. They also have a toll-free telephone hot-line service staffed by professionals that provides information about all aspects of the prevention and treatment of asthma. If the person who answers the phone cannot answer your question, you will be contacted by a member of the staff who can.

RECOMMENDED READING

Asthma by Allan M. Weinstein, M.D. (New York: Fawcett Crest, 1988, 357 pp., $4.95)

This is the best, most comprehensive book available to the general public on adult asthma. In addition to detailed, up-to-date information about the disease, Dr. Weinstein offers a comprehensive self-care program for asthma patients.

Children with Asthma: A Manual for Parents by Thomas F. Plaut, M.D. (Amherst, Mass.: Pedipress, 1984, 271 pp., $11.95) (Available for $13.95 postpaid from Pedipress, 125 Red Gate Road, Amherst, Mass. 01002)

The finest and most complete book available about asthma and children. Contains much information about diagnosis and treatment of childhood asthma as well as numerous sources for materials, treatment, and support.

Breathing Easy by Genell Subak-Sharpe (New York: Doubleday, 1988, 250 pp., $17.95)

A fine book describing the treatment program of the National Jewish Center for Immunology and Respiratory Medicine.

The Essential Asthma Book by François Haas, Ph.D., and Sheila Sperber Haas, Ph.D. (New York: Ivy Books, 1987, 362 pp., $4.95)

A very comprehensive book about all aspects of asthma.

The Asthma Handbook by Stuart H. Young, M.D., with Susan A. Shulman and Martin D. Shulman, Ph.D. (New York: Bantam Books, 1989, 366 pp., $9.95)

Another comprehensive and informative asthma book for both children and adults.

Who Gets Sick? by Blair Justice, Ph.D. (Los Angeles: Jeremy P. Tarcher, Inc., 1988, 407 pp., $17.95)

This important book explores how our beliefs, moods, and thoughts can affect our health. While not written specifically for asthma patients, it includes the latest medical findings on the power of the mind to enhance health and diminish disease.

Love Your Disease by John Harrison, M.D. (Santa Monica, Calif.: Hay House, 1989, 285 pp., $9.95).

Although not specifically about asthma, this interesting book, written by an Australian physician and therapist, examines the psychological basis for disease. He also offers an innovative approach to self-healing.

INDEX

ABOUT THE AUTHORS

NATHANIEL ALTMAN has been writing about health and psychological topics for more than twenty years. He is a graduate of the University of Wisconsin and the author of over a dozen books, including *Eating for Life* (Quest) and *Everybody's Guide to Chiropractic Health Care* (Jeremy P. Tarcher). Mr. Altman lives in Brooklyn, N.Y.

DAVID A. MRAZEK, M.D., M.R.C. Psych., has been director of pediatric psychiatry at the National Jewish Center for Immunology and Respiratory Medicine in Denver for more than a decade. He is also an associate professor of child psychiatry and pediatrics at the University of Colorado School of Medicine in Denver, Colorado.